Men's Fitness
GUIDE TO BUILDING A
COVER MODEL BODY

By **Joe Warner**

Art Editor Richard Davis
Designer Fanni Williams
Photography Tom Miles, Duncan Nicholls
Models Kirk Miller, Oliver Jedrej@WAthletic
Subeditor Chris Miller

For more information on *Men's Fitness* magazine go to **mensfitness.co.uk**

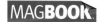

Group Publisher **Russell Blackman**
Digital Production Manager **Nicky Baker**
MagBook Publisher **Dharmesh Mistry**
Operations Director **Robin Ryan**
Managing Director of Advertising
Julian Lloyd-Evans
Newstrade Director **David Barker**
Commercial & Retail Director **Martin Belson**
Chief Operating Officer/
Chief Financial Officer **Brett Reynolds**
Group Finance Director **Ian Leggett**
Chief Executive Officer **James Tye**
Chairman **Felix Dennis**

The 'MagBook' brand is a trademark of Dennis Publishing Ltd,
30 Cleveland Street, London W1T 4JD. Company registered in England.
All material © Dennis Publishing Ltd, licensed by Felden 2012,
and may not be reproduced in whole or part without the
consent of the publishers. Printed at BGP Bicester.

MEN'S FITNESS GUIDE TO BUILDING
A COVER MODEL BODY ISBN 1-78106-017-7
To license this product please contact Nicole Adams on
+44 (0) 20 7907 6134 or email nicole_adams@dennis.co.uk

Advertising
Katie Wood katie_wood@dennis.co.uk
Matt Wakefield matt_wakefield@dennis.co.uk

To subscribe to *Men's Fitness* magazine, call **0844 844 0081** or go to **mensfitness.co.uk**

Contents

Introduction

Cover model workouts

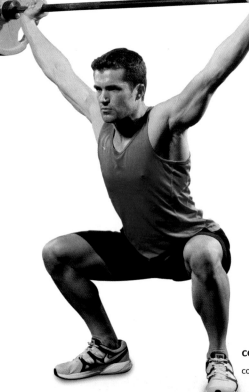

COMPOUND GAINS
Performing heavy
compound lifts is the
best way to build a
cover model body

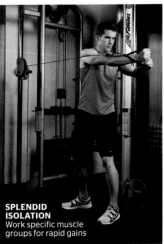

**SPLENDID
ISOLATION**
Work specific muscle
groups for rapid gains

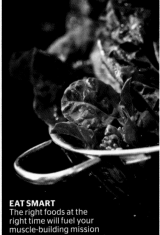

EAT SMART
The right foods at the
right time will fuel your
muscle-building mission

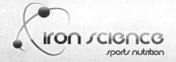
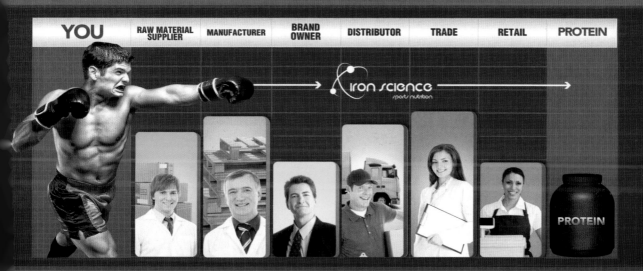
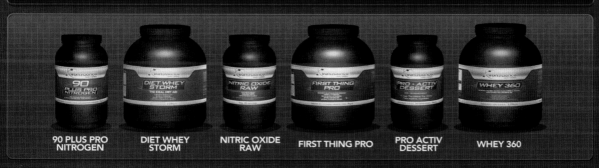

CHANGE

TO A SUPERIOR PROTEIN

Instant Whey is unlike other whey proteins and the differences can deliver you significant benefits.

166% more bio available cystine, 16% more leucine
It uses Native Whey which is different to conventional whey protein having a less invasive pasteurising process. As a result it contains up to 166% more bio available cystine than conventional whey which is vital for optimal immune function and therefore recovery after exercise. It also contains up to 16% more leucine which helps to build and repair muscle.

It is unbeaten in terms of its protein levels at a guaranteed level of 80%. Containing a market leading protein percentage also means that it contains less fat and less carbohydrate.

Given our unique approach to quality we are able to offer a simple, no questions asked Full Money Back Guarantee (see website).

If you haven't tried Instant Whey recently, you owe it to yourself to do so. Not only is it unique in respect of the inclusion of Native Whey, market leading in terms of its protein percentage but it also comes in a range of fantastic flavours and is covered by a simple and effective guarantee.

This explains why we are inviting you to change to a superior protein.

Protein percentage		Cost per g of protein
Reflex Instant Whey inc. Native Whey	**80%**	**3.3p**
Competitor brand A	78.5%	3.5p
Competitor brand B	78%	3.37p
Competitor brand C	76.6%	4.32p
Competitor brand D	72%	3.57p
Competitor brand E	70%	3.75p

Delivering such a high quality product can only be achieved by controlling the entire manufacturing process and testing each batch produced. Not only does Reflex operate what is arguably the most advanced manufacturing unit in the UK but every single batch of Instant Whey is protein tested and the results published on our website.

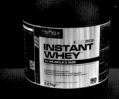

**Instant Whey™
inc. Native Whey**
Part of our High Protein range

Find out more about our products at:

www.reflex-nutrition.com

 Please visit & join our Facebook page at Reflex Nutrition Ltd

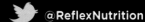 @ReflexNutrition

ecotricity

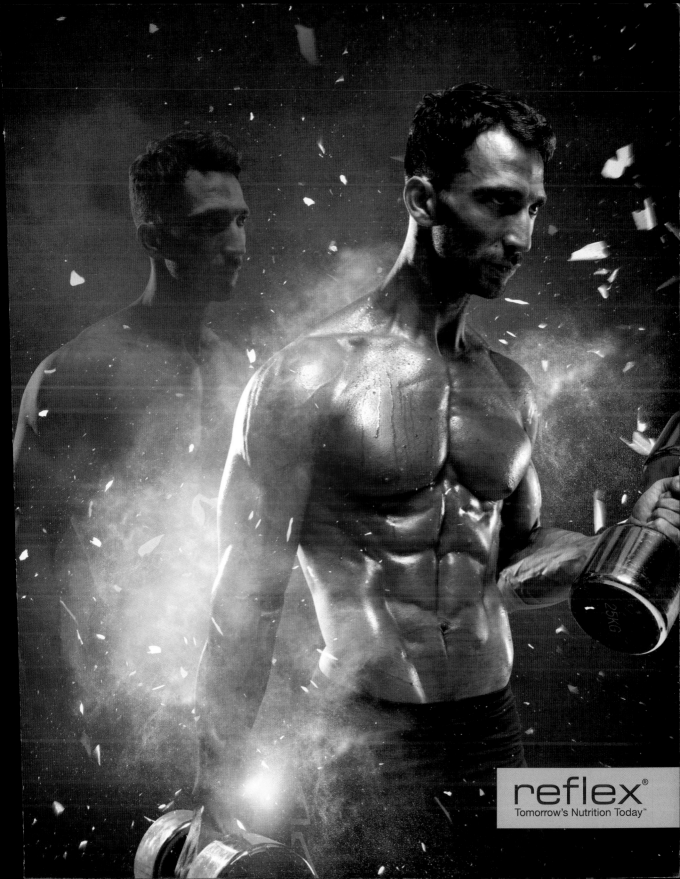

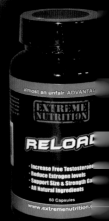
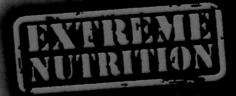
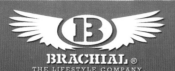

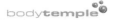

About this book

Build a body even a *Men's Fitness* magazine cover model would be proud of

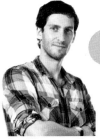

Joe Warner, editor

Here at *Men's Fitness* we ask a lot from the models who we meet at castings when trying to find the right man to grace our cover.

All of them have a strong, lean and athletic body but that's not enough. We only choose those select few who, through weeks, months and even years of hard graft, have built a body that will inspire our tens of thousands of readers into getting up off the sofa and making a positive change to the way they look and feel for a healthier, happier and more successful life.

We know that many of you want to look just like our cover stars, which is why we have written this book. It's the definitive guide to building big muscles where you most want them in the quickest and most efficient way possible.

Muscle mission

The book is divided into nine chapters. We start by explaining how your muscles work and how to prepare them for exercise. The next six chapters focus on how to add size and strength to specific muscle groups: your arms, abs, chest, shoulders, back and legs. Chapter eight is based around total-body exercises, which is a great way to add even more muscle while getting all the fat-burning benefits of working multiple muscle groups in a single session. The result? You look even more ripped with your shirt off.

The final chapter details exactly what you need to eat and why to make gains fast while burning fat, along with a comprehensive guide to the supplements that can make your muscle-building mission even easier.

Ready? Let's go!

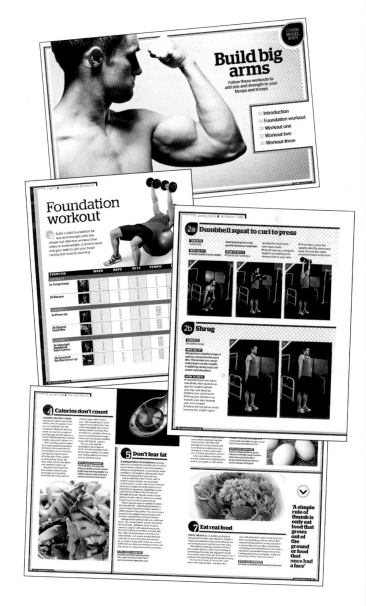

Muscle Q&A

No-nonsense answers to the fundamental fitness questions

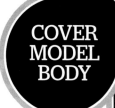

Q I've failed to add muscle in the past. Why will it work now?

A If your efforts have been unsuccessful in the past, this had nothing to do with your body being fundamentally resistant to exercise and everything to do with your approach. In other words, you didn't have a focused plan, didn't set realistic, achievable goals or didn't eat the right foods – or some combination of the three. Anyone can make positive changes to the way they look, but that's not going to happen overnight. Going to the gym once or twice a week won't give you a radical transformation, especially if you don't work hard or aren't eating well.

Q Can I turn my body fat into muscle?

A Fat and muscle are two totally different types of tissue so it's impossible for one to turn into the other. Muscle is active tissue that burns calories, while fat tissue stores excess energy. When you train hard you burn away fat and build muscle, giving an appearance that one has turned into the other, but this is not the case.

Q How often do I need to work out?

A Less frequently than you might think. And it's certainly not the case that more is better.

That's because it's actually when you're recovering that your muscle size and strength increases. If you don't take the time to recover sufficiently you won't see improvements. It's not just your muscles that need time to recover; your nervous system is working hard to recruit your muscles, something it's not used to doing, so it also needs time to recover.

Q How long should each workout last?

A The perfect workout should take less than an hour to complete, including warm-up, warm-down and stretching. Research suggests that your levels of the growth hormone testosterone peak around 45 minutes into a workout and then quickly subside as your levels of cortisol, the stress hormone that breaks down muscle tissue and damages cells, rise. So keep your workouts short and effective.

Q Do crunches build a six-pack?

A You can perform hundreds of crunches every day and have the strongest abs in the world, but if they're under a layer of fat then you're not going to see them. And if you're trying to burn fat, crunches are just about the worst move you could choose. In fact, you'd have to do about 500,000 of them to burn

1kg of fat. That's about four weeks of nonstop crunching.

Q Are machines better than free weights?

A Resistance machines have their place in a gym: they're a great way for beginners to learn movement patterns without the risk of injury, and they allow experienced trainers to isolate specific muscles to lift more weight. But because the movement is restricted, they won't work the stabilising muscles that are so important in keeping you free of injury. Using free weights may require more skill, but it will recruit those stabilising muscles and better prepare your body for other activities, especially sports.

Q How quickly will I see results?

A Even with the help of this book, don't expect overnight success. You need to lift heavy weights regularly to stimulate the muscle into growing, eat a diet of high-quality protein and carbs with no junk and get plenty of sleep. It's a big commitment.

Q Aren't squats bad for my knees?

A Performed incorrectly, any move is dangerous, although squats have a

particularly bad reputation. But a correct squat – in which your feet are shoulder-width apart and your knees stay in line with your toes – places emphasis on the quads, glutes and hamstrings, and not on any joints. This can reduce the risk of injury by strengthening the muscles and supporting tissues around the knee joint.

Q Are lighter weights best for toning?

A 'Toning' is one of the most popular words in the exercise world. It is also one of the most redundant. You can't 'tone' a muscle, only build it or maintain it, while stripping away fat to give it a more prominent appearance. So when people say they want to 'tone up' they actually mean that they want to add muscle, lose fat or a bit of both.

FIT TIP
It's best to have a check-up with a GP before you begin training.

Q How effective are bodyweight moves?

A If you're new to training or returning from injury, bodyweight moves are the perfect preparation for heavier lifts. They can also be used effectively as part of supersets or bodyweight circuits, and are far better at building strength and stability in your joints and core than resistance machines.

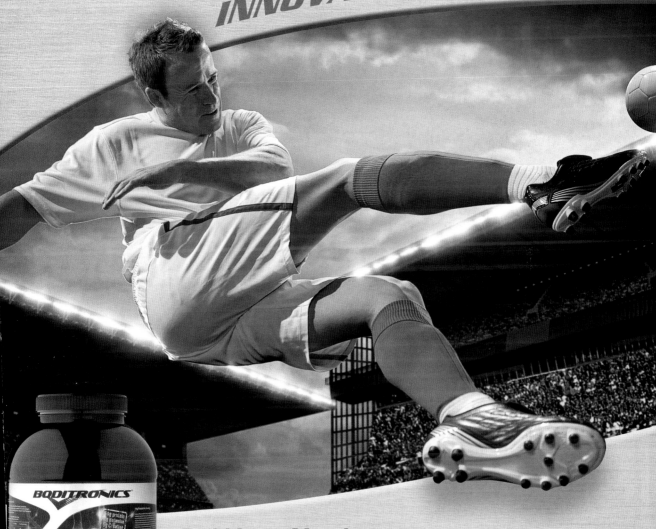

BODITRONICS®

INNOVATION IN ACTION

Build Lean Muscle...

EXPRESS WHEY ANABOLIC

- Contains 54g Protein, 5g Creatine per serving
- First and only protein to include D Aspartic Acid for muscle growth, increased, power, strength, endurance and recovery
- A superior muscle building protein
- Delivers results fast.

www.boditronics.co.uk

Growth targets

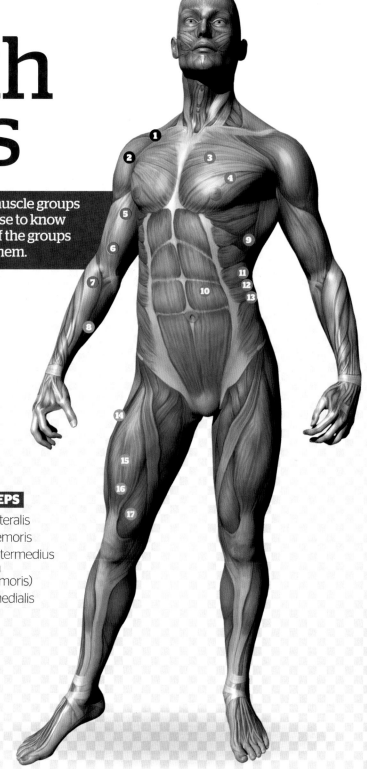

You're going to target all the major muscle groups in this workout plan, so it makes sense to know what they are. Here are the names of the groups and the individual muscles within them.

DELTOIDS
1 Medial deltoid (middle)
2 Anterior deltoid (front)

PECTORALS
3 Pectoralis major
4 Pectoralis minor (beneath the pectoralis major)

BICEPS
5 Biceps brachii
6 Brachialis
7 Brachioradialis

FOREARMS
8 Flexor carpi radialis

ABDOMINALS
9 Serratus anterior
10 Rectus abdominis
11 External obliques
12 Internal obliques (beneath external obliques)
13 Transverse abdominis (beneath internal obliques)

QUADRICEPS
14 Vastus lateralis
15 Rectus femoris
16 Vastus intermedius (beneath rectus femoris)
17 Vastus medialis

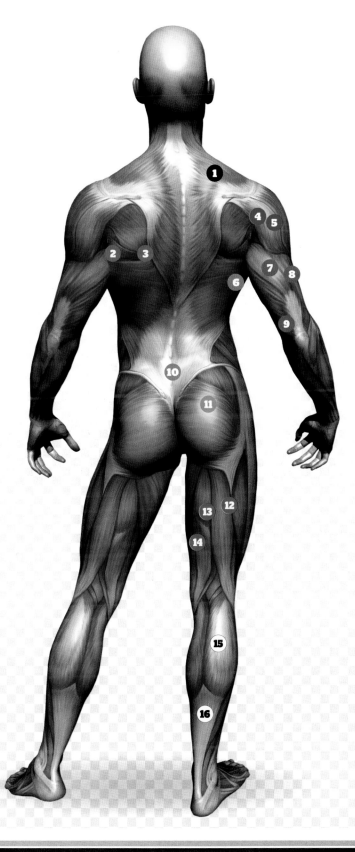

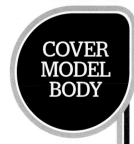

TRAPS

1 Trapezius

BACK

2 Teres major
3 Rhomboid (beneath trapezius)

DELTOIDS

4 Rotator cuff (beneath deltoids)
5 Posterior deltoid (back)

LATS

6 Latissimus dorsi

TRICEPS

7 Triceps brachii long head
8 Triceps brachii lateral head
9 Triceps brachii medial head

LOWER BACK

10 Erector spinae

GLUTES

11 Gluteus maximus

HAMSTRINGS

12 Biceps femoris
13 Semitendinosus
14 Semimembranosus

CALVES

15 Gastrocnemius
16 Soleus

Pre-workout warm-up

Do this routine before every workout to prepare your body and prevent injury

A proper warm-up is vital before doing any weight training. If time is short, don't be tempted to skip the warm-up and go straight to your workout, because cold muscles can get easily damaged. Saving a few minutes saved on a warm-up can mean losing days to injury.

Your warm-up should start with some light cardiovascular exercise, such as running, rowing or cycling. This will make your heart beat faster, pumping oxygen and nutrients to your muscles and elevating your body's core temperature. Warm muscles are more elastic than cold ones, which allows you to work them through a greater range of motion with less injury risk.

After the cardio you need to target your muscles directly with dynamic stretches. These differ from static stretches in that you are moving as you stretch the muscle. The trick is to start very gently and then slowly increase the range of motion you go through with each repetition. This prepares your muscles and joints for the work to come.

Finally, before you begin any lifting exercise, perform the movement with minimal weight to teach your muscles how to respond when you do the exercise with full weights.

Cardio
10 MINUTES

Whatever method of cardio warm-up you choose, keep the pace gentle and constant. By the end of ten minutes you should be sweating and puffing a bit, but not out of breath.

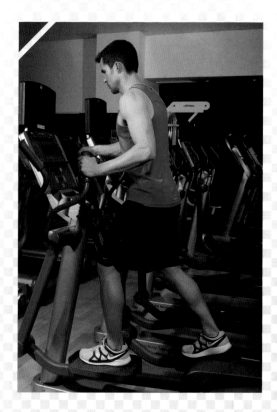

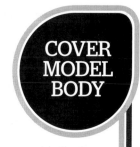
Dynamic stretches
10 REPS OF EACH

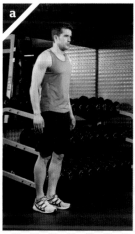
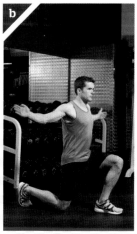

1 Lunge with reverse flye
- Step forward while stretching your arms to the sides
- Keep your body upright
- Lunge lower with each rep

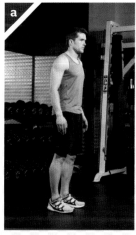
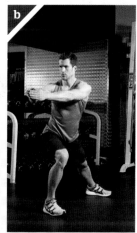

2 Lateral lunge with twist
- Step to the side with both feet pointing forwards
- Twist your torso in the direction of your leading foot
- Bend your knee a bit further with each rep

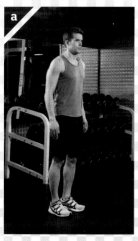
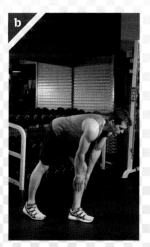

3 Alternating split deadlift
- Step forward with one foot and lean forwards at the hips, then push back to the start
- Keep your back straight
- Lower your hands down your shins a bit further each time

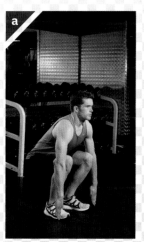
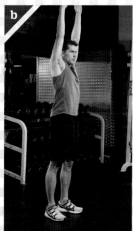

4 Squat to overhead reach
- Start with your feet shoulder-width apart and back straight
- Squat down, then reach overhead as you stand up
- Squat a bit lower with each rep

Post-workout stretches

Ease your tired muscles after every workout

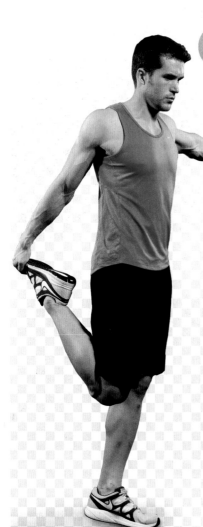

A static stretch is when you hold a muscle under tension while relaxing it in order to lengthen the muscle after it has contracted as a result of weight training. Performing static stretches after a workout provides several benefits.

First, it will help with flexibility, so you'll be able to work your muscles across a greater range of motion, leading to better muscle gains. Stretching also helps reduce injuries because your muscles and tendons are less likely to tear when they are relaxed.

Stretching improves blood flow to your muscles, helping to flush out toxins, which means you'll be ready for your next workout sooner. And stretching can also aid posture because tense muscles can pull your spine, shoulders and hips out of alignment, leading to a stooped look and lower-back pain.

It's important for your muscles to be fully warmed up before you perform static stretches, so never do them before your workout – save them for afterwards.

Static stretches
Hold each for 20 to 30 seconds

To avoid injury, don't pull too hard when you stretch your muscles, and never 'bounce' the muscle under tension. Always maintain control throughout.

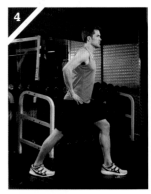

Calves
● Push down on your rear heel

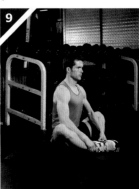

Adductors
● Press your knees apart gently with your elbows

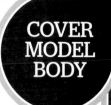
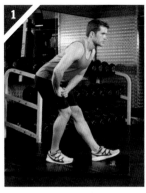

Hamstrings
- Lean forward at the hips with a straight back

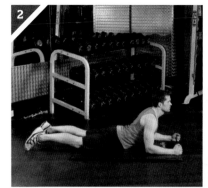

Abs
- Lift your shoulders high off the floor

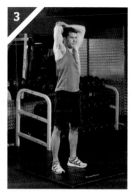

Triceps
- Point fingers downwards and pull your elbow gently

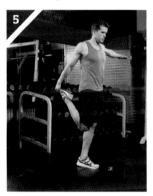

Quads
- Pull on your ankle and push your hips forward

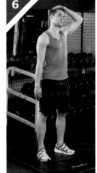

Traps
- Pull gently on your head

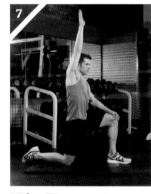

Hip flexors
- Keep your body upright and push your hips forwards

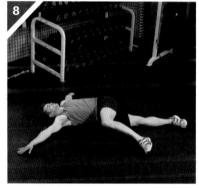

Lower back
- Keep your shoulders flat on the floor

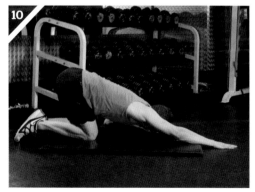

Lats
- Press your shoulders towards the floor

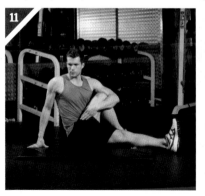

Glutes
- Gently pull on your knee

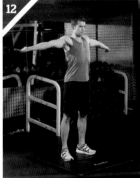

Biceps
- Press your arms back and point your thumbs behind you

Cover model under construction

How this plan will transform your body in under a month

The aim of the plan is simple: to burn body fat and build muscle as quickly as possible. To achieve that goal, all the workouts in this book are based on a training method called German Body Composition, a protocol designed by *MF*'s muscle expert Charles Poliquin, a strength and conditioning coach who has trained Olympians in 12 sports as well as leading professional sportsman in the NFL, NHL and English Premier League. The protocol is so effective because it combines heavy strength training with short rest breaks, so you not only get the muscle-building benefits of lifting, but also the fat-burning benefits of high-intensity training. Here's the deal.

Workout design

Each workout is made up of three supersets: two exercises performed back to back without rest. The three main workouts in each chapter begin with a superset of two compound moves – exercises that work more than one muscle group – while the second two involve exercises that isolate specific muscle groups to elicit the greatest growth response. The foundation workout at the start of each chapter also

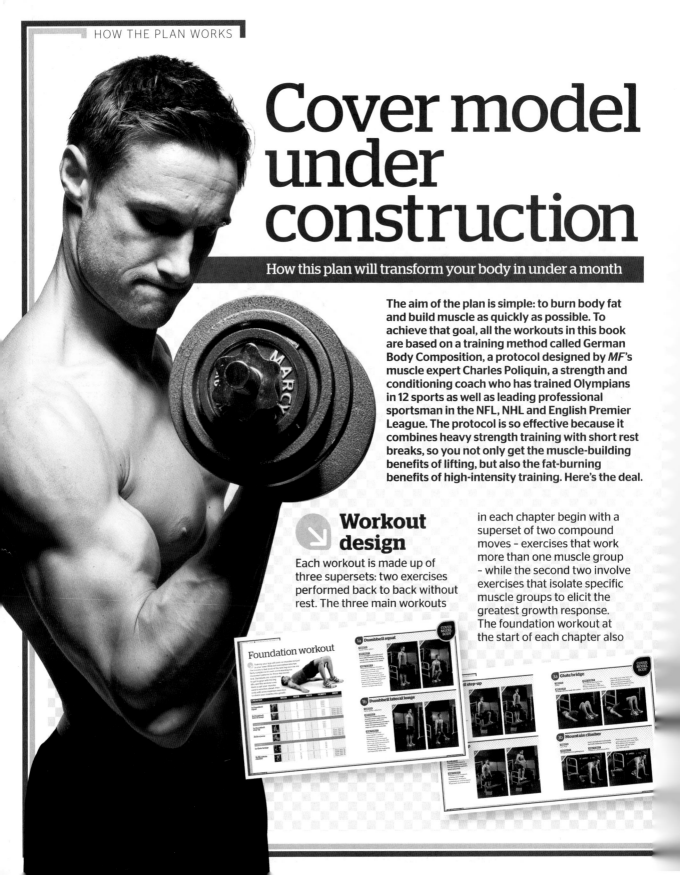

Workout theory

Each routine is shown in table form. Here's how the tables work

WEEK

Four weeks isn't long enough for your body to get so comfortable with the exercises that it stops responding. This means you can do the same moves each week and get great results, particularly if you're adjusting other variables such as sets, rest and tempo. And by sticking with the same moves for three weeks you'll get better at the movement patterns involved in each exercise so you'll be able to lift heavier each week.

REPS

This is the number of times you perform an exercise in each set. All the rep counts are designed to result in hypertrophy (muscle growth) but they are not all the same because not all muscle groups respond in the same way. Muscle groups with higher numbers of type 2 muscle fibres (the ones responsible for fast, explosive movements) respond better to lower rep ranges than muscle groups made up of more type 1 muscle fibres (those responsible for endurance efforts).

SETS

For each workout in the first week you perform two sets of the prescribed number of reps. This is because they're new workouts so your body needs to get used to the movements, and that's demanding. Once you're more familiar with the moves you can increase the set count.

TEMPO

This refers to the speed of the lift. If you want to see the best results, it's vital that you stick to the right tempo for every part of the lift. The first number is the speed in seconds of the lowering portion of a lift, such as lowering the bar to your chest in a bench press. The second is the pause at the bottom, the third is the speed of lifting the weight and the fourth is the pause between reps. An X means that you should do that part of the move as quickly as possible.

REST

This is the amount of time you should take between supersets. You should aim not to rest between the two exercises in a superset, then rest for the allotted time between supersets. Rest for two to three minutes between groups of supersets. The rest time is reduced from week two onwards to make the workout more challenging and the rest times have been picked to maximise growth hormone release.

EXERCISE		WEEK	REPS	SETS	TEMPO	REST
SUPERSET 1						
1a Front squat		1	10	2	20X0	
		2	8	3	20X0	
		3	8	3	30X0	
		4	10	4	30X0	
1b Sumo deadlift		1	10	2	20X0	90sec after 1b
		2	8	3	20X0	90sec after 1b
		3	10	3	20X0	90sec after 1b
		4	8	4	20X0	90sec after 1b
SUPERSET 2						
2a Push press		1	10	2	30X0	
		2	8	3	30X0	
		3	8	3	40X0	
		4	10	4	30X0	
2b Tuck jump		1	12	2	X	90sec after 2b
		2	10	3	X	75sec after 2b
		3	12	3	X	75sec after 2b
		4	12	4	X	90sec after 2b
SUPERSET 3						
3a Single-leg calf raise		1	12	2	2111	
		2	12	3	2111	
		3	15	3	2111	
		4	12	4	2111	
3b Dumbbell step-up		1	12	2	1111	90sec after 3b
		2	12	3	1111	75sec after 3b
		3	15	3	1111	60sec after 3b
		4	12	4	1111	60sec after 3b

contains compound moves, but is more focused on isolation exercises that hit the target muscle group to build up your strength levels.

Why are supersets so effective?

Doing supersets reduces the amount of time you spend resting during a workout, which ensures that the intensity of the session remains high. The two compound move supersets pair either upper-body and lower-body exercises or those that work opposite (or antagonistic) muscle groups. This means you can lift heavy weights for both moves because while one set of muscles is working, the others are recovering. With this method you are able to sustain a very high effort level, or intensity, which will torch calories.

The next four moves focus on specific muscle groups to fully fatigue them, which shocks your body into growing them back bigger and stronger.

What weight should I use?

Pick a weight that means you struggle to complete the final couple of reps of the last set. This is likely to mean that you need to use a weight that is at least 70% of your one-repetition maximum – the weight you can only lift once with perfect form.

What should I eat?

Good news. You don't have to follow a restrictive diet. The key things are to eat fresh food, make sure you are eating high levels of protein and avoiding refined carbohydrates such as white bread, rice and pasta. You'll find the nutrition rules you should live by on p162.

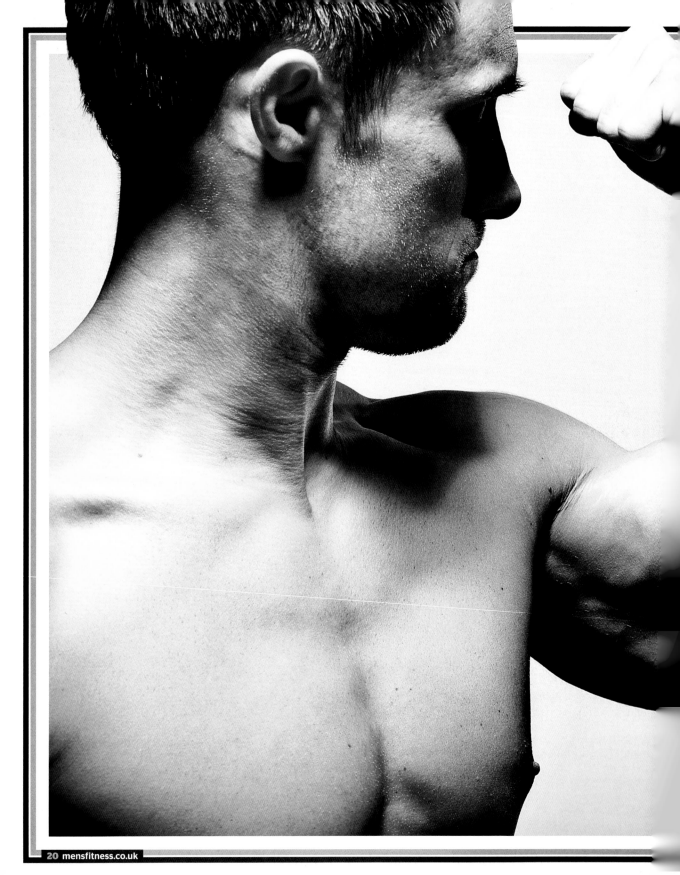

Build big arms

Follow these workouts to add size and strength to your biceps and triceps

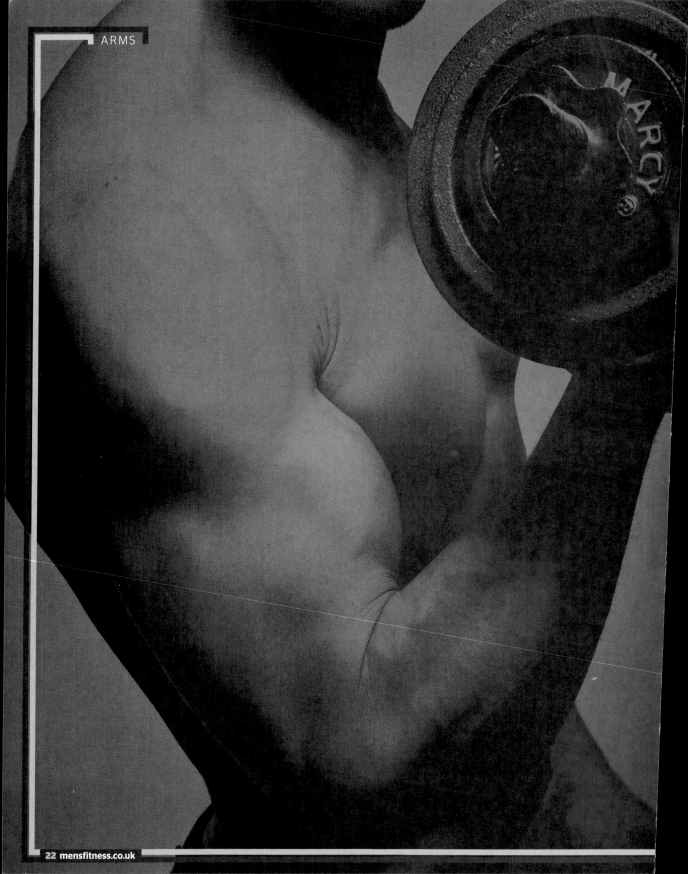

Win the arms race

Let's face it. Every guy wants impressive arms. Ones that fill the sleeves of a T-shirt. That's why many men spend hours banging out hundreds of reps of biceps curls in an attempt to get huge guns. Problem is, that's not the best way. All you'll get is sore muscles and smug looks from everyone else in the gym. Here's all you need to know.

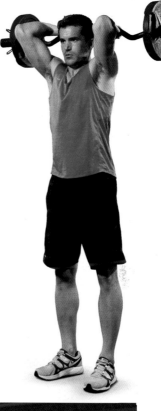

How to do the workouts
Make gains fast with these four muscle-specific training plans

There are four workouts in this chapter. Each of these programmes is based on doing three sessions per week for a total of four weeks.

The first plan is a foundation workout designed for men of all athletic abilities, so make sure you start off by following this one rather than jumping straight into one of the three main workouts.

For those of you new to this type of exercise it will build a solid base from which you can launch into the more intense workouts. And even if you are a more experienced trainer, there's still much to gain from starting with the basics. It will help correct any muscular imbalances you may have, allow you to correct any poor form habits you may have picked up and let you master some simple movement patterns, including bodyweight moves, that you may have neglected during most of your previous training regimes.

ANATOMY OF THE MUSCLE GROUP ARMS

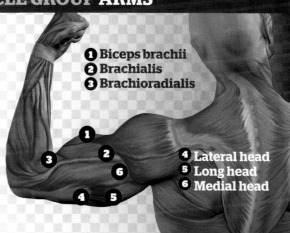

Biceps
The biceps is made up of three muscle sections. The biceps brachii is a two-part muscle that bends and lifts your arm. It is supported by the brachialis, which is recruited when your palms are facing downwards. This, in turn, is aided by the brachioradialis, which sits mainly on the forearm but is involved in flexing the elbow.

Triceps
The triceps, as the name suggests, is made up of three 'heads' – lateral, long and medial – and it makes up about two-thirds of your upper arm muscle. The lateral and medial heads of the triceps are involved in straightening your arm, while the long head is engaged when you draw your arms down in front of you.

1 Biceps brachii
2 Brachialis
3 Brachioradialis

4 Lateral head
5 Long head
6 Medial head

Foundation workout

This workout is designed with three aims in mind: to get your heart-rate high to improve cardiovascular fitness; to get your biceps and triceps used to movement patterns involved in many of the moves that directly work the arms; and to build a good foundation layer of strength so that you can attack the three main workouts right from the gun.

EXERCISE		WEEK	REPS	SETS	TEMPO	REST
SUPERSET 1						
1a Bodyweight squat		1 2 3 4	10 12 10 12	2 2 3 3	2010 2010 2010 2010	
1b Press-up burpee		1 2 3 4	8 10 8 10	2 2 3 3	X X X X	90sec after 1b 90sec after 1b 90sec after 1b 90sec after 1b
SUPERSET 2						
2a Dumbbell hammer curl		1 2 3 4	10 12 10 12	2 2 3 3	3010 3010 3010 3010	
2b Reverse-grip dumbbell row		1 2 3 4	10 12 10 12	2 2 3 3	2010 2010 2010 2010	90sec after 2b 90sec after 2b 90sec after 2b 90sec after 2b
SUPERSET 3						
3a Diamond press-up		1 2 3 4	8 10 8 10	2 2 3 3	2010 2010 2010 2010	
3b Bench dip		1 2 3 4	10 12 10 12	2 2 3 3	2010 2010 2010 2010	90sec after 3b 90sec after 3b 90sec after 3b 90sec after 3b

1a Bodyweight squat

TARGETS
Glutes, quads, hamstrings

WHY DO IT?
Mastering the correct form of
a bodyweight squat means
you'll make quicker progress
when adding additional weight
through a barbell or dumb-bell.

HOW TO DO IT
● Stand with your feet
shoulder-width apart and
pointing out slightly.
● Keeping your core braced
and a natural arch in your back,
squat down until your thighs are
parallel to the floor, then push
back up through your heels.

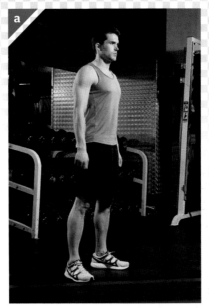
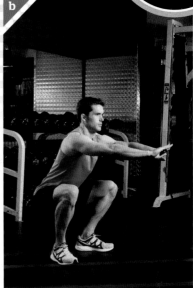

1b Press-up burpee

TARGETS
Total body

WHY DO IT?
This is a great move for working
multiple muscle groups at
once. It will get your heart
rate soaring and really fire up
your upper-body muscles.

HOW TO DO IT
● Start standing with your
arms fully extended above
your head, then squat down.
● As you reach the bottom of
the squat, put your hands on
the ground in front of you and
kick your legs backwards until
you are in a press-up position.
● Perform a press-up, then bring
your legs back underneath you
and jump up off the ground.

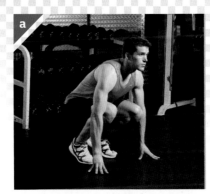
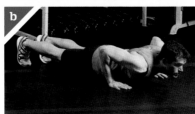
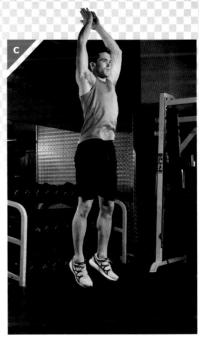

2a Dumbbell hammer curl

TARGETS
Biceps

WHY DO IT?
This move works your forearms for improved grip strength, as well as your biceps.

HOW TO DO IT
● Stand tall with your shoulders back and feet close together, holding a dumbbell in each hand with your palms facing each other.
● Keeping your elbows close to your sides, slowly raise the dumbbells up to shoulder height, squeezing your biceps at the top of the move.
● Slowly return the weight to the start position.

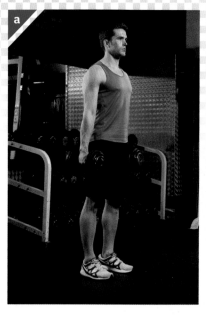
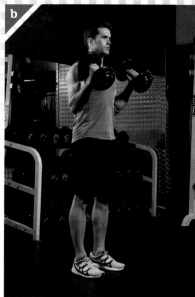

2b Reverse-grip dumbbell row

TARGET
Biceps, upper back

WHY DO IT?
This move works your biceps as well as the powerhouse muscles of your upper back.

HOW TO DO IT
● Hold a dumbbell in each hand with arms fully extended and lean forwards from the hips, keeping your back straight.
● Row the weights up towards your chest, then slowly return to the start position.

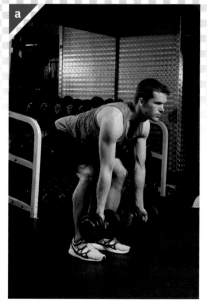
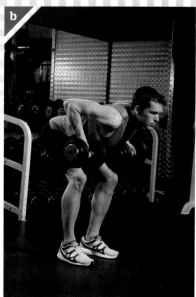

3a Diamond press-up

TARGETS
Triceps, chest

WHY DO IT?
Having your hands close together shifts the focus away from the chest towards your triceps.

HOW TO DO IT
● Start in a press-up position but with your hands close together so that opposite thumbs and index fingers touch to form a diamond.
● Keeping your body in a straight line from head to heels, lower as far as you can.
● Press back up strongly to the start position.

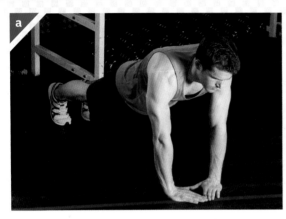

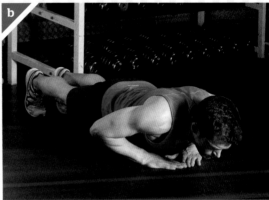

3b Bench dip

TARGET
Triceps

WHY DO IT?
It works your triceps without forcing you to lift your entire bodyweight. Bend your knees to make it easier; straighten your legs to make it harder.

HOW TO DO IT
● Place your hands on the edge of a bench behind you with your back and legs straight.
● Slowly lower your body straight down, keeping your elbows pointing back throughout, then press back up powerfully.

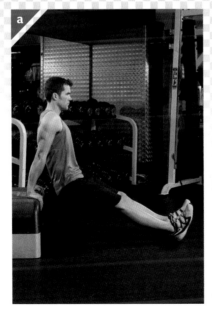

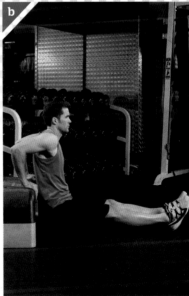

Workout one

Kicking off with two of the best big lifts for packing size on to your lower and upper body, this session then moves on to hit first the biceps and then the triceps hard with back-to-back moves. The first superset primes your muscles for growth by releasing testosterone and other growth hormones, which are shuttled towards your arms during the final four moves.

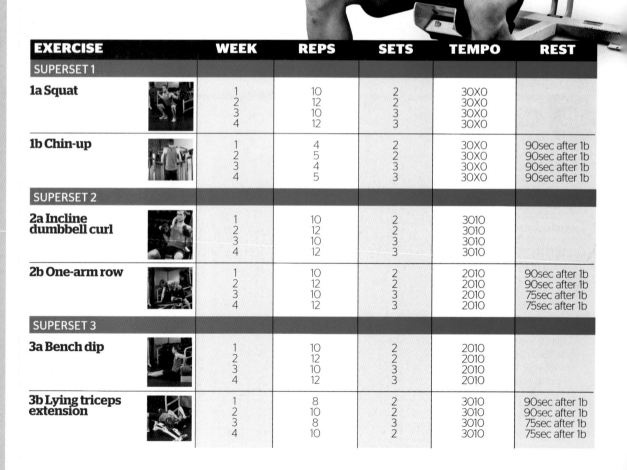

EXERCISE		WEEK	REPS	SETS	TEMPO	REST
SUPERSET 1						
1a Squat		1 2 3 4	10 12 10 12	2 2 3 3	30X0 30X0 30X0 30X0	
1b Chin-up		1 2 3 4	4 5 4 5	2 2 3 3	30X0 30X0 30X0 30X0	90sec after 1b 90sec after 1b 90sec after 1b 90sec after 1b
SUPERSET 2						
2a Incline dumbbell curl		1 2 3 4	10 12 10 12	2 2 3 3	3010 3010 3010 3010	
2b One-arm row		1 2 3 4	10 12 10 12	2 2 3 3	2010 2010 2010 2010	90sec after 1b 90sec after 1b 75sec after 1b 75sec after 1b
SUPERSET 3						
3a Bench dip		1 2 3 4	10 12 10 12	2 2 3 3	2010 2010 2010 2010	
3b Lying triceps extension		1 2 3 4	8 10 8 10	2 2 3 2	3010 3010 3010 3010	90sec after 1b 90sec after 1b 75sec after 1b 75sec after 1b

1a Squat

TARGETS
Quads, glutes, hamstrings

WHY DO IT?
Heavy lifts trigger the release of testosterone and growth hormone so you get bigger everywhere.

HOW TO DO IT
- Rest the bar against the back of your shoulders, holding it with an overhand grip. Both your hands and your feet should be just wider than shoulder-width apart.
- Lower yourself – keeping your chest up – until your thighs are at least parallel to the floor. The deeper you can squat, the better.
- Drive back up through your heels without letting your knees roll inwards.

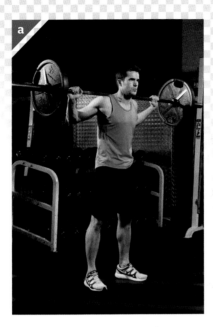
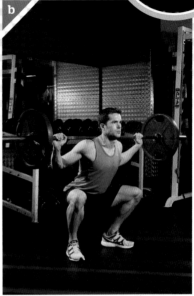

1b Chin-up

TARGETS
Biceps, upper back, core

WHY DO IT?
It's a safe way of really challenging your back and biceps muscles.

HOW TO DO IT
- Grasp the bars with an underhand grip. If using a straight bar your hands should be shoulder-width apart.
- Start from a dead hang with your arms fully extended.
- Pull yourself up by squeezing your lats together.
- Once your chin is higher than your hands pause briefly, then slowly lower yourself back to the start until your arms are fully extended.

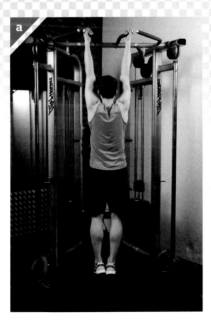
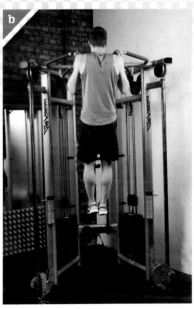

2a Incline dumbbell curl

TARGETS
Biceps

WHY DO IT?
Performing biceps curls on an incline bench allows you to move through a greater range of motion than doing them standing up, so they have to work harder.

HOW TO DO IT
● Sit on a bench set on an incline between 30˚ and 45˚ holding a dumbbell in each hand.
● Keeping your back flat against the bench and your elbows close to your sides, slowly curl one dumbbell up to shoulder height.
● Squeeze your biceps at the top of the move before slowly returning the start and repeating with your other arm.

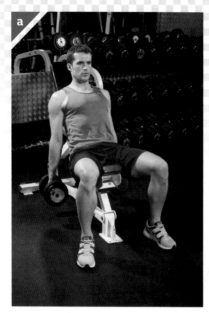
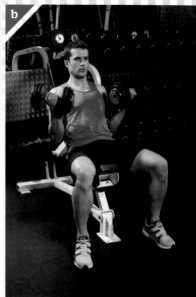

2b One-arm row

TARGETS
Biceps, upper back

WHY DO IT?
Working each arm individually prevents you from relying on your stronger side, resulting in balanced gains.

HOW TO DO IT
● Place your left knee and left hand flat on a bench, with your right foot flat on the ground beside it. Hold a dumbbell in your right hand.
● With a natural arch in your back and core braced, lift the weight up towards your side, leading with the elbow.
● Slowly return the weight back to the start and repeat on the other side.

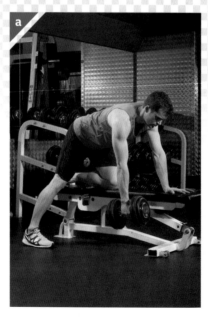
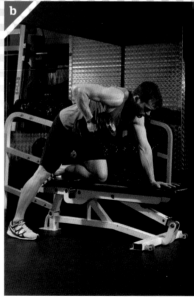

3a Bench dip

TARGETS
Triceps

WHY DO IT?
Build muscular strength on the back of your arms with this bodyweight move. Keep your legs straight to make it harder.

HOW TO DO IT
● Place your hands on the edge of a bench behind you with your back and legs straight.
● Slowly lower your body straight down, keeping your elbows pointing back throughout, before pressing back up powerfully.

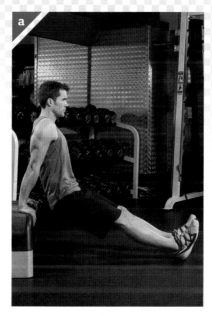
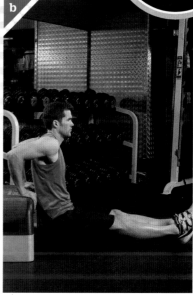

3b Lying triceps extension

TARGETS
Triceps

WHY DO IT?
This move isolates your triceps, forcing them to work hard throughout the entire move to lower the weight under control and raise it again.

HOW TO DO IT
● Lie flat on a bench, holding an EZ-bar above you with straight arms.
● Slowly lower the bar towards the top of your head by bending your elbows, which should stay pointing directly up.
● Without arching your back, slowly return the bar to the start position by straightening your arms.

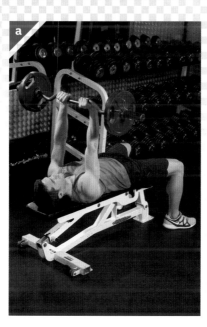
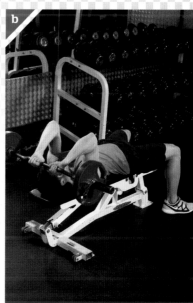

Workout two

The deadlift is the single best move for promoting an anabolic (muscle-building) state in your body. Pairing it with a variation on the classic bench press, which shifts the focus on to your triceps, creates a great superset to start the second of your three arms workouts. You'll then hit your arms hard for rapid results.

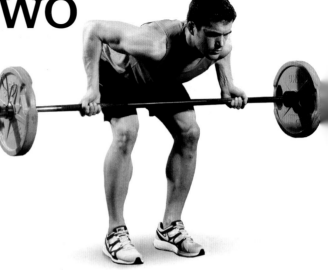

EXERCISE		WEEK	REPS	SETS	TEMPO	REST
SUPERSET 1						
1a Deadlift		1	8	2	20X0	
		2	10	2	20X0	
		3	8	3	20X0	
		4	10	4	20X0	
1b Close-grip bench press		1	8	2	40X0	90sec after 1b
		2	10	2	40X0	90sec after 1b
		3	8	3	40X0	90sec after 1b
		4	10	4	40X0	90sec after 1b
SUPERSET 2						
2a Reverse-grip bent-over row		1	8	2	2010	
		2	10	2	2010	
		3	8	3	2010	
		4	10	4	2010	
2b Standing cable row		1	10	2	2010	75sec after 2b
		2	12	2	2010	75sec after 2b
		3	10	3	2010	75sec after 2b
		4	12	4	2010	75sec after 2b
SUPERSET 3						
3a Standing triceps extension		1	10	2	2010	
		2	12	2	2010	
		3	10	3	2010	
		4	12	4	2010	
3b Medicine ball press up		1	10	2	2010	75sec after 3b
		2	12	2	2010	75sec after 3b
		3	10	3	2010	75sec after 3b
		4	12	4	2010	75sec after 3b

1a Deadlift

TARGETS
Total body

WHY DO IT?
It may not work your arms directly but you can't afford to ignore the overall muscle-building benefits of this classic lift.

HOW TO DO IT
- Grip the bar just outside your knees with your core braced, your shoulders retracted and over the bar and your back flat.
- Use your glutes to power the initial lift, pushing down through your heels.
- Keep the bar close to your body and, as it passes your knees, push your hips forward. Keep your shoulders back throughout the move.

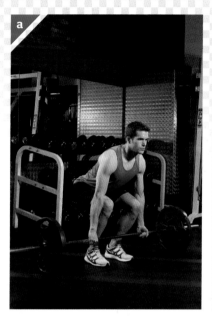
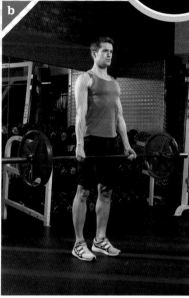

1b Close-grip bench press

TARGETS
Triceps, chest

WHY DO IT?
Bringing your hands close together transfers the focus of this move from the chest and to the triceps.

HOW TO DO IT
- Lie flat on a bench holding a barbell with an overhand grip and a fist-sized gap between your hands.
- Keep your core braced and feet flat on the floor.
- Lower the bar slowly to your chest, keeping your elbows close your sides to keep the emphasis on your triceps.
- Push back up powerfully, but don't lock out your elbows.

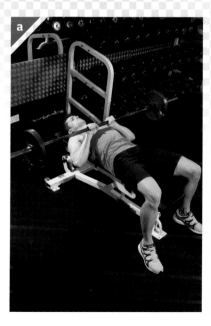
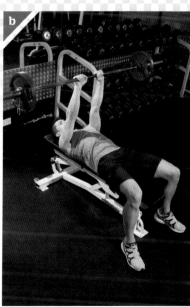

2a Reverse-grip bent-over row

TARGETS
Biceps, upper back

WHY DO IT?
The bent-over row works the powerhouse muscles of the upper back and the reverse grip places greater emphasis on your biceps. Your abs are also involved to keep your torso stable.

HOW TO DO IT
● Start with your core braced and your back straight. Bend your knees slightly and lean forwards from the hips.
● Hold the bar with an underhand grip with your hands just wider than shoulder-width apart.
● Pull the bar up almost to your chest, retracting your shoulder blades, then lower it slowly to the start.

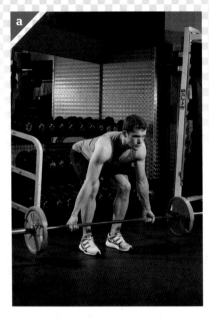
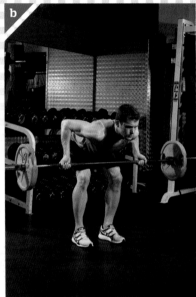

2b Standing cable row

TARGETS
Biceps, upper back

WHY DO IT?
This move works your biceps as well as the muscles of your upper back.

HOW TO DO IT
● Stand tall at a cable machine with a handle attached at about bellybutton height.
● Hold a handle in each hand and step backwards so that there is tension in the cable.
● Keeping your body still, pull the handles in to your stomach, leading with your elbows so that they stay close to your sides.
● Return to the start.

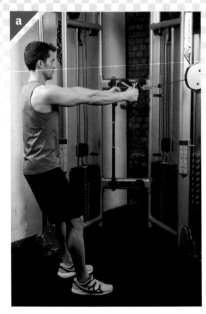
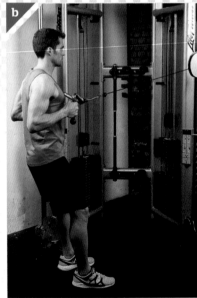

3a Standing triceps extension

TARGETS
Triceps

WHY DO IT?
This move isolates your triceps, forcing them to work hard throughout the entire move to control the weight down then back up again.

HOW TO DO IT
● Stand tall, holding an EZ-bar above you with straight arms.
● Slowly lower the bar towards the back of your head by bending your elbows, which should stay pointing directly up.
● Without arching your back, slowly return the bar to the start position by straightening your arms.

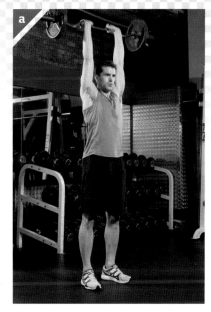
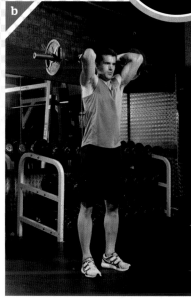

3b Gym ball press-up

TARGETS
Triceps, chest

WHY DO IT?
This press-up variation places greater emphasis on the triceps, while the instability of the ball forces your core to work overtime.

HOW TO DO IT
● Start in a press-up position with your hands on a gym ball.
● Keeping your body in a straight line from head to heels, lower your chest until it touches the ball, then press back up strongly.

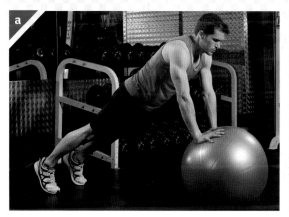
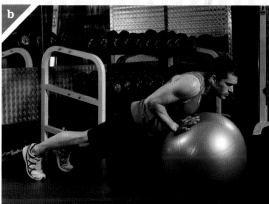

Workout three

This final workout is the hardest, hitting your muscles with compound lifts that work all your major muscle groups to burn fat and build muscle mass. The result is not just bigger arms – it's also greater size and strength across your entire torso, helping to create that cover model look.

EXERCISE		WEEK	REPS	SETS	TEMPO	REST
SUPERSET 1						
1a Pull-up		1 2 3 4	6 8 6 8	2 3 3 4	30X0 30X0 30X0 30X0	
1b Clean and press		1 2 3 4	8 10 8 10	2 3 3 4	X X X X	90sec after 1b 90sec after 1b 90sec after 1b 90sec after 1b
SUPERSET 2						
2a EZ-bar curl		1 2 3 4	10 10 12 10	2 3 3 4	20X0 20X0 20X0 20X0	
2b Upright row		1 2 3 4	8 8 10 8	2 3 3 4	20X0 20X0 20X0 20X0	90sec after 2b 90sec after 2b 90sec after 2b 90sec after 2b
SUPERSET 3						
3a Dip		1 2 3 4	10 8 10 8	2 3 3 4	30X0 30X0 30X0 30X0	
3b Seated dumbbell shoulder press		1 2 3 4	12 10 12 10	2 3 3 4	20X0 20X0 20X0 20X0	90sec after 3b 90sec after 3b 90sec after 3b 90sec after 3b

1a Pull-up

TARGETS
Upper back, core

WHY DO IT?
This is a seriously tough move because you control and lift your entire weight in conflict with gravity, but it'll build a strong, wide upper back, which helps create a wide, V-shaped torso.

HOW TO DO IT
- Grasp the bars with an overhand grip. If using a straight bar, your hands should be slightly wider than shoulder-width apart.
- Start from a dead hang with your arms fully extended.
- Pull yourself up by squeezing your lats together.
- Once your chin is higher than your hands, pause and then return to the start.

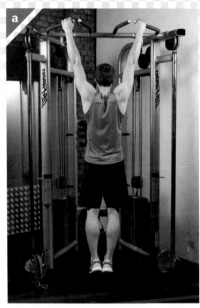
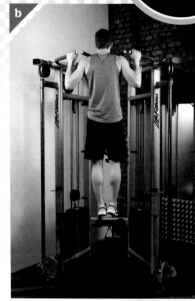

1b Clean and press

TARGETS
Total body

WHY DO IT?
The clean involves almost all your major muscle groups, forcing them to work together efficiently.

HOW TO DO IT
- Squat down and hold the bar with an overhand grip.
- Lift the bar by driving through your heels.
- Once the bar reaches your hips, rise onto your toes and shrug your shoulders to pull the bar higher, leading with your elbows.
- When it's at shoulder height, squat and rotate your elbows forward to catch the bar on your shoulders, then press it directly overhead.

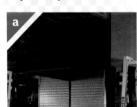
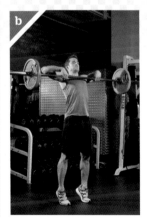
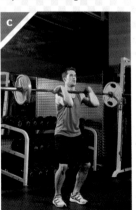
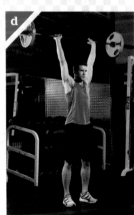

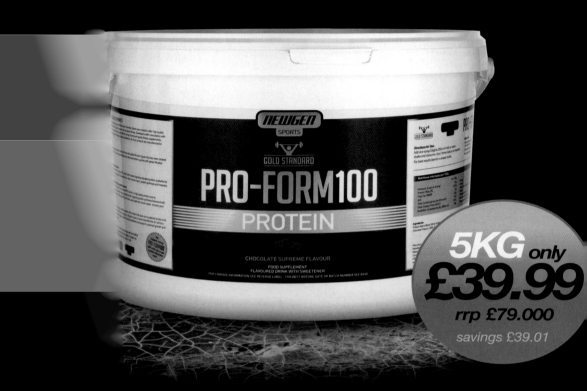

2a | EZ-bar biceps curl

TARGETS
Biceps

WHY DO IT?
Using an EZ-bar, which has a zigzagged middle, allows you turn your hands inwards slightly. This places the focus solely on your biceps, forcing them to work hard throughout the move.

HOW TO DO IT
- Stand tall with your shoulders back and feet close together, holding an EZ-bar with an underhand grip with hands just outside your hips.
- Keeping your elbows tucked in to your sides, curl the bar up towards your chest.
- Lower back slowly to the start.

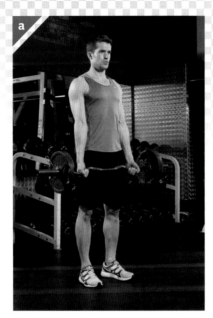
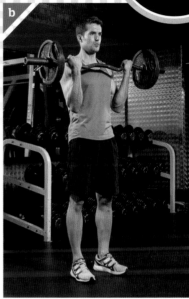

2b | Upright row

TARGETS
Biceps, shoulders

WHY DO IT?
Although this move mainly works your traps and shoulders, getting a strong upper back will assist with the 'shrugging' part of the main snatch lift, helping you generate sufficient power to lift the bar up and over your head.

HOW TO DO IT
- Stand tall, holding a barbell with an overhand grip slightly narrower than shoulder-width.
- Shrug the bar up towards your chin, leading with your elbows, which should point upwards.
- Slowly lower the bar back to the start.

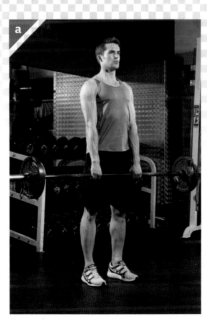
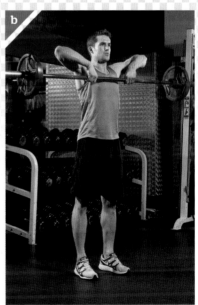

3a Triceps dip

TARGETS
Triceps, lower chest, shoulders

WHY DO IT?
Dips are one of the best moves for targeting all three parts of the triceps, as well as working the lower chest, shoulders and core, which you must keep tight to prevent your lower body swinging.

HOW TO DO IT
● Grip parallel bars, keeping your body upright.
● With your elbows pointing straight back, lower your body as far as you can comfortably go without stressing your shoulders.
● Keep your core braced and don't swing your legs for momentum.

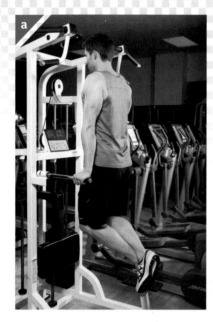
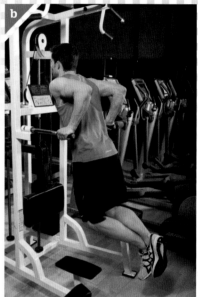

3b Seated dumbbell shoulder press

TARGETS
Shoulders, triceps

WHY DO IT?
Performing this move seated means you can lift heavier to really hit your shoulders and triceps.

HOW TO DO IT
● Sit on an upright bench holding a dumbbell in each hand at shoulder height.
● Keep your feet flat on the floor, core braced, back against the bench and head looking forward.
● Press the weights up powerfully until your arms are fully extended, then return slowly to the start.

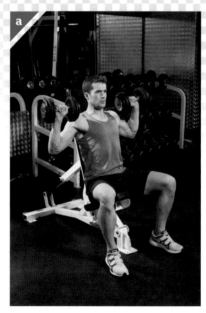
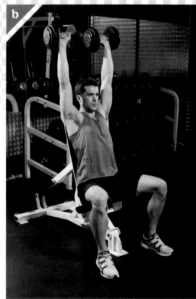

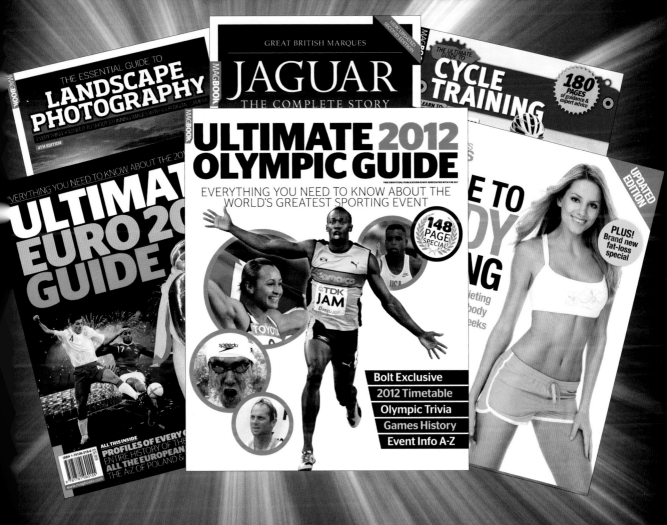

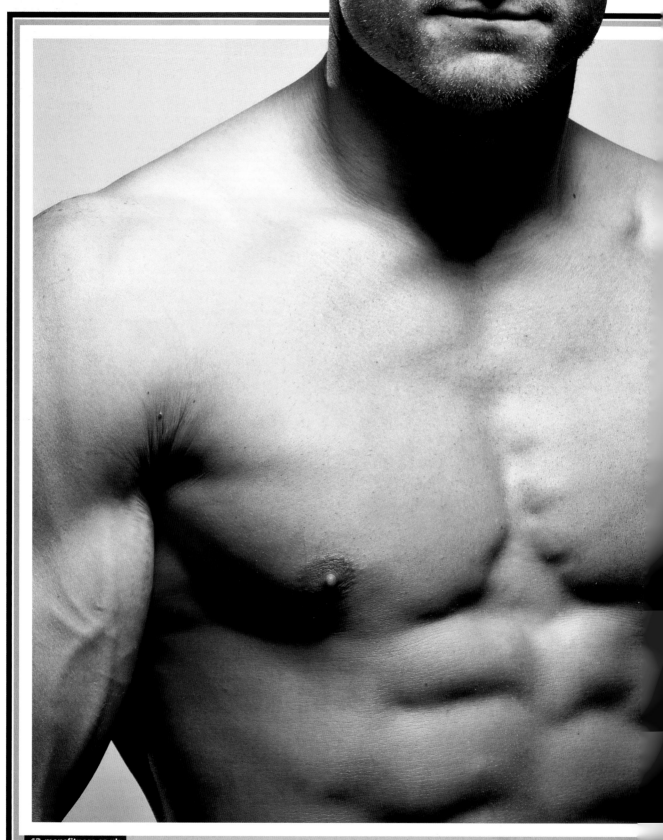

Get a huge chest

Sculpt powerful pecs in no time with these no-nonsense workouts

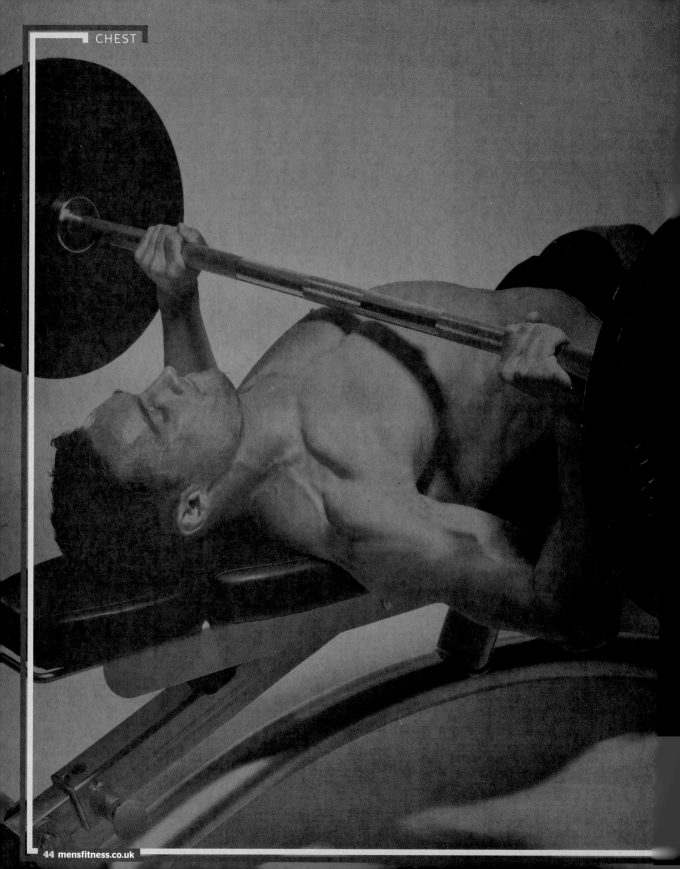

Get pecs appeal

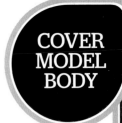
To build a strong and powerful chest you need to do far more than crank out rep after rep on the bench press. Don't get us wrong, it is a hugely important lift to add size to your chest, but it alone won't sculpt the muscles you want. Here's what will.

How to do the workouts
Make gains fast with these four muscle-specific training plans

There are four workouts in this chapter. Each of these programmes is based on doing three sessions per week for a total of four weeks.

The first plan is a foundation workout designed for men of all athletic abilities, so make sure you start off by following this one rather than jumping straight into one of the three main workouts.

For those of you new to this type of exercise it will build a solid base from which you can launch into the more intense workouts. And even if you are a more experienced trainer, there's still much to gain from starting with the basics. It will help correct any muscular imbalances you may have, allow you to

correct any poor form habits you may have picked up and let you master some simple movement patterns, including bodyweight moves, that you may have neglected during most of your previous training regimes.

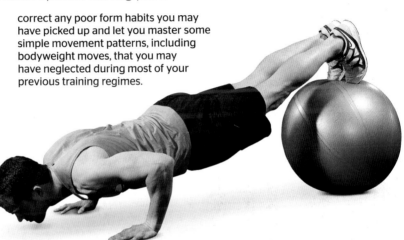

ANATOMY OF THE MUSCLE GROUP CHEST

The main job of the pecs is to push your arms in front of you, and they are also used when bringing your arms down in front of you. There are two main muscles in this group.

Pectoralis major

The pectoralis major is a large muscle that attaches to your collarbone, breastbone and ribs. Although it is a single muscle, most experienced weight trainers divide the chest into three portions: upper, middle and lower. Any chest exercise will work the entire pectoralis

major, but by varying the angle – by doing incline or decline bench presses – it is possible to target the upper or lower parts of the chest.

Pectoralis minor

The pectoralis minor is a thin triangular muscle found near the shoulder and below the pectoralis major. The function of the pectoralis minor is to bring the shoulder forward, an important part of generating strength in big chest moves.

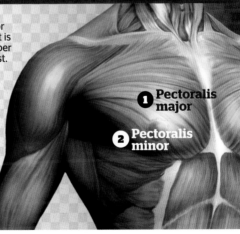

1 Pectoralis major

2 Pectoralis minor

Foundation workout

Build a solid foundation for size and strength with this simple but effective workout that relies on bodyweight, a stretch band and gym balls to get your heart racing and muscles burning.

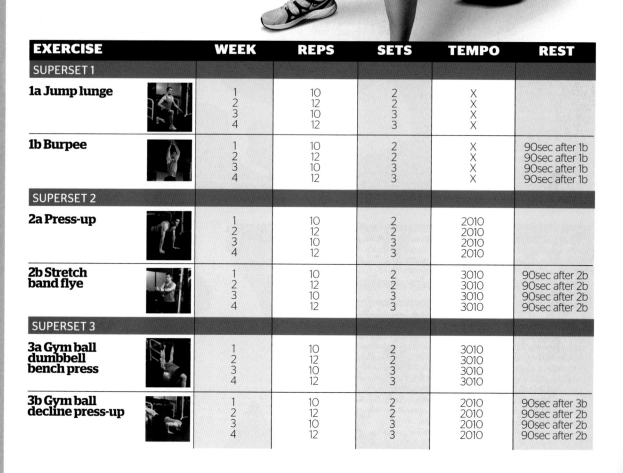

EXERCISE		WEEK	REPS	SETS	TEMPO	REST
SUPERSET 1						
1a Jump lunge		1	10	2	X	
		2	12	2	X	
		3	10	3	X	
		4	12	3	X	
1b Burpee		1	10	2	X	90sec after 1b
		2	12	2	X	90sec after 1b
		3	10	3	X	90sec after 1b
		4	12	3	X	90sec after 1b
SUPERSET 2						
2a Press-up		1	10	2	2010	
		2	12	2	2010	
		3	10	3	2010	
		4	12	3	2010	
2b Stretch band flye		1	10	2	3010	90sec after 2b
		2	12	2	3010	90sec after 2b
		3	10	3	3010	90sec after 2b
		4	12	3	3010	90sec after 2b
SUPERSET 3						
3a Gym ball dumbbell bench press		1	10	2	3010	
		2	12	2	3010	
		3	10	3	3010	
		4	12	3	3010	
3b Gym ball decline press-up		1	10	2	2010	90sec after 3b
		2	12	2	2010	90sec after 2b
		3	10	3	2010	90sec after 2b
		4	12	3	2010	90sec after 2b

1a Jump lunge

TARGETS
Quads, hamstrings, glutes

WHY DO IT?
Adding a jump turns this classic bodyweight exercise into a powerful plyometric move that fires up your fast-twitch muscles fibres and gets your heart rate pumping.

HOW TO DO IT
● Stand with one foot forward and bend both knees to about 90˚, then jump powerfully up into the air, switching legs in mid-air.
● Land with the other foot forward and lower into another lunge, then repeat.

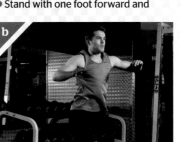
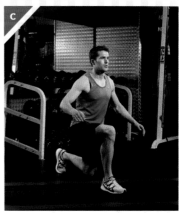

1b Burpee

TARGETS
Total body

WHY DO IT?
This is a great move for working multiple muscle groups at once.

HOW TO DO IT
● Stand with your feet shoulder-width apart, then lower into a squat.
● As you reach the bottom of the squat, put your hands on the ground and kick your legs back until you are in a press-up position.
● Bring your legs back underneath you, then jump up off the ground.

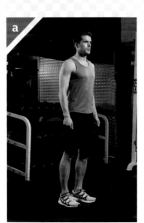
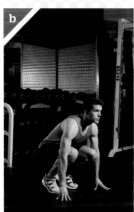
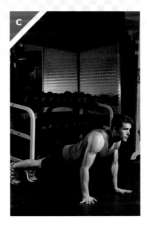
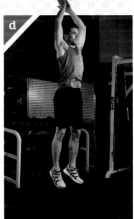

2a Press-up

TARGETS
Chest, triceps

WHY DO IT?
Press-ups require your chest, shoulder, triceps and core muscles to work hard to lower, then lift, your torso.

HOW TO DO IT
● Start with your hands shoulder-width apart and body straight.
● Lower yourself until your elbows reach 90°, then press back up.

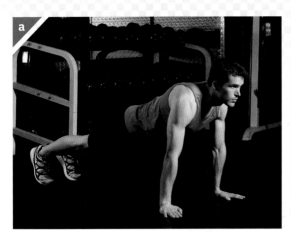
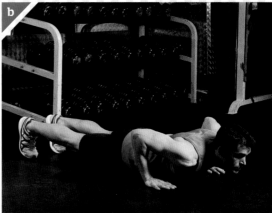

2b Stretch band flye

TARGETS
Chest

WHY DO IT?
This is a great way to work the chest without the need for weights, and the constant tension of the band works your muscles through every rep.

HOW TO DO IT
● Run a stretch band around a fixed object then turn so your back is to it, holding one end in each hand with arms out to the sides.
● Maintaining a slight bend in your elbow, bring your arms out and around in a semi-circle so that your hands meet in front of your body.
● Slowly return to the start.

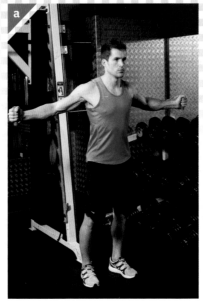
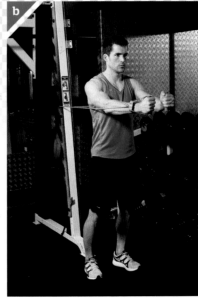

3a Gym ball dumbbell bench press

TARGETS
Chest, triceps

WHY DO IT?
The instability of the ball makes your core work hard to stabilise your torso during each rep.

HOW TO DO IT
● Lie with your upper back supported on a gym ball and your arms extended above you, holding a dumbbell in each hand.
● Slowly lower the weights down towards your chest, then press back up powerfully.

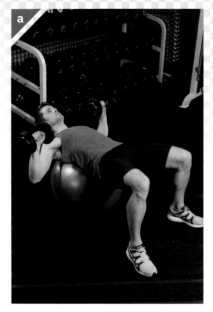
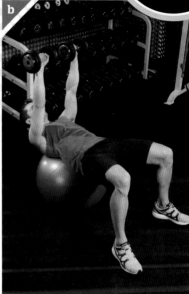

3b Gym ball decline press-up

TARGETS
Chest, triceps, shoulders

WHY DO IT?
Having your feet on the ball makes your core work hard and works the lower part of your chest.

HOW TO DO IT
● Start with both feet on a gym ball and your hands on the floor underneath your shoulders.
● Keeping your core braced, bend your elbows to lower your chest to the floor, then press back up.

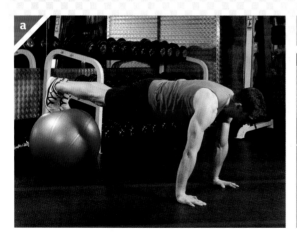
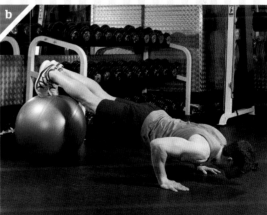

Workout one

This workout begins with two tough supersets, designed to alternately work your chest and the major muscles of the upper back. This ensures your growth is balanced and reduces the risk of injury. It finishes with two surprisingly tough bodyweight moves to really blitz your chest before you can hit the showers.

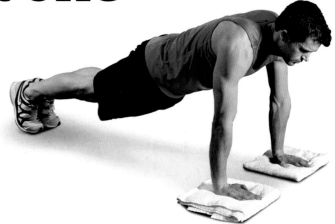

EXERCISE		WEEK	REPS	SETS	TEMPO	REST
SUPERSET 1						
1a Bench press		1	8	2	4010	
		2	10	2	4010	
		3	8	3	4010	
		4	10	3	4010	
1b Bent-over row		1	8	2	2010	90sec after 1b
		2	10	2	2010	90sec after 1b
		3	8	3	2010	90sec after 1b
		4	10	3	2010	90sec after 1b
SUPERSET 2						
2a Incline dumbbell flye		1	10	2	3010	
		2	12	2	3010	
		3	10	3	3010	
		4	12	3	3010	
2b Dumbbell pullover		1	10	2	3010	90sec after 2b
		2	12	2	3010	90sec after 2b
		3	10	3	3010	90sec after 2b
		4	12	3	3010	90sec after 2b
SUPERSET 3						
3a Press-up		1	10	2	2010	
		2	12	2	2010	
		3	10	3	2010	
		4	12	3	2010	
3b Towel flye slide		1	10	2	2010	90sec after 3b
		2	12	2	2010	90sec after 3b
		3	10	3	2010	90sec after 3b
		4	12	3	2010	90sec after 3b

1a Bench press

TARGETS
Chest, triceps, shoulders

WHY DO IT?
This classic lift works the chest plus the muscles at the front of the shoulders and the back of the arms, making it a firm favourite for those wanting a big, strong torso.

HOW TO DO IT
● Lie flat on a bench with your core braced, your shoulder blades retracted and your feet underneath your knees.
● Holding a barbell with an overhand grip, slowly lower the bar down towards your nipples.
● Press back up powerfully to straighten your arms but don't lock out your elbows.

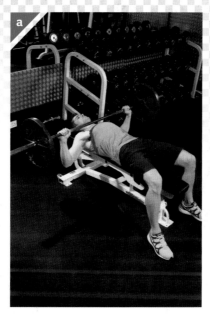
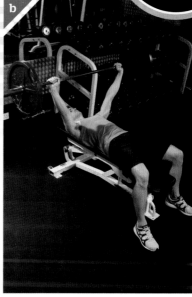

1b Bent-over row

TARGETS
Upper back, biceps

WHY DO IT?
It works the opposite muscle group to the bench press, giving you balanced upper-body strength to prevent muscular imbalance and injury.

HOW TO DO IT
● Start with your core braced, your back straight and your shoulder blades retracted.
● Bend your knees slightly and lean forward from the hips.
● Grip the bar with your hands just wider than shoulder-width apart.
● Pull the bar up almost to your chest, retracting your shoulder blades, then lower it slowly to the start.

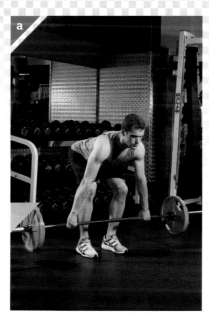
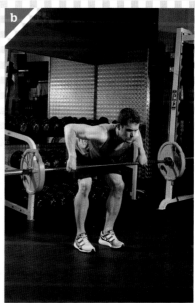

2a Incline dumbbell flye

TARGETS
Chest

WHY DO IT?
This move isolates your chest muscles, which means all the work is done by the chest.

HOW TO DO IT
● Lie on an incline bench holding a dumb-bell in each hand directly above your chest with palms facing.
● Make sure your head and shoulders are supported and that your feet are flat on the floor.
● Keeping a slight bend in your elbows, slowly lower the weights out to the sides as far as is comfortable. Don't arch your back.
● Use your pecs to reverse the movement to raise the weights back to the top.

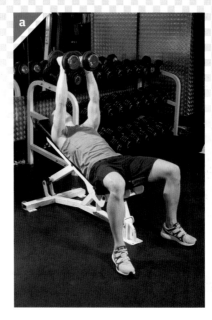
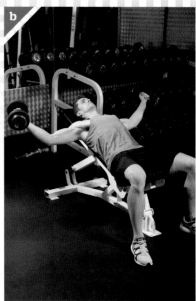

2b Dumbbell pullover

TARGETS
Chest, shoulders, upper back

WHY DO IT?
It works your lower chest, back and triceps at once.

HOW TO DO IT
● Lie flat on a bench with head and shoulders supported and feet flat.
● Hold a single dumb-bell with both hands over your chest.
● Slowly lower the weight behind your head then use your pecs to pull it back to the start position.

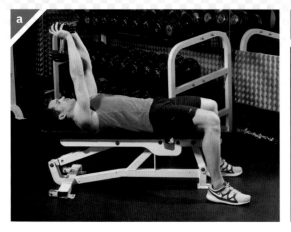
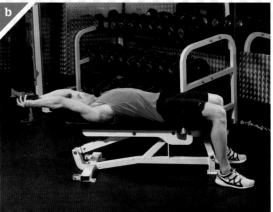

3a Press-up

TARGETS
Chest, triceps

WHY DO IT?
The ultimate upper-body test, press-ups require your chest, shoulder, triceps and core muscles to work hard to lower, then lift your torso to the floor.

HOW TO DO IT
● Start with your hands shoulder-width apart and body straight.
● Lower yourself until your elbows reach 90˚, then press back up.

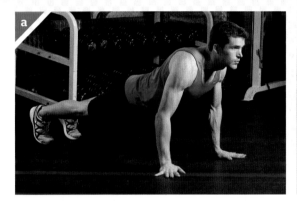
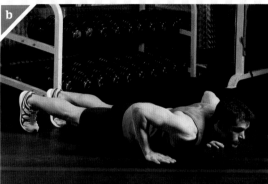

3b Towel flye slide

TARGETS
Chest, shoulders, core

WHY DO IT?
This moves works the chest through a wide range of motion.

HOW TO DO IT
● Start in a press-up position with your hands on top of small towels.
● Slowly slide your arms out to the sides so that your chest is lowered toward the floor.
● Once your arms are wide, reverse the movement to the start.

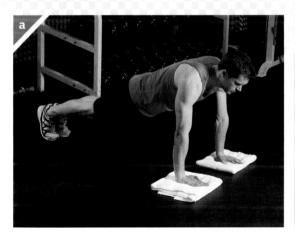
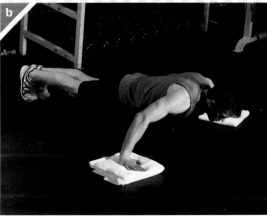

Workout two

Starting with two big moves to work your legs, shoulders, triceps and chest will fire up your central nervous system to elicit the best growth-hormone response for the rest of the workout, which focuses on the chest and abs to forge a solid torso.

EXERCISE		WEEK	REPS	SETS	TEMPO	REST
SUPERSET 1						
1a Push press		1 2 3 4	10 12 10 10	2 2 3 4	30X0 30X0 30X0 30X0	
1b Decline bench press		1 2 3 4	8 10 8 8	2 2 3 4	40X0 40X0 40X0 40X0	90sec after 1b 75sec after 1b 90sec after 1b 90sec after 1b
SUPERSET 2						
2a Incline dumbbell press		1 2 3 4	10 12 10 10	2 2 3 4	30X0 30X0 30X0 30X0	
2b Cable crossover		1 2 3 4	10 12 12 12	2 2 3 4	20X0 20X0 20X0 20X0	90sec after 2b 75sec after 2b 90sec after 2b 90sec after 2b
SUPERSET 3						
3a T press-up		1 2 3 4	10 12 10 10	2 2 3 4	X X X X	
3b Plank		1 2 3 4	1 1 1 1	2 2 3 4	30sec 45sec 45sec 30sec	90sec after 3b 75sec after 3b 90sec after 3b 90sec after 3b

1a Push press

TARGETS
Legs, core, shoulders

WHY DO IT?
Using your legs to assist the move allows you to lift heavier, priming your muscles for growth.

HOW TO DO IT
● Stand with feet shoulder-width apart with the bar resting across the front of your shoulders.
● Bend your knees slightly, then stand up straight to generate momentum. As you do, press the bar directly overhead.
● Slowly lower the weight back to the start position.

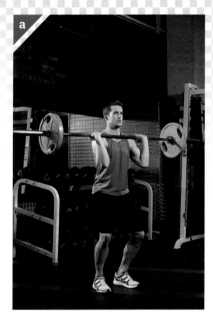
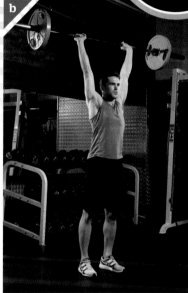

1b Decline bench press

TARGETS
Chest, shoulders, triceps

WHY DO IT?
Varying the classic chest move by using a decline bench shifts some of the focus towards the lower part of your pec muscles.

HOW TO DO IT
● Lie on a decline bench with your feet on the floor, with your head, upper back and glutes should be flat against the bench.
● Hold the bar with an overhand grip that is wider than shoulder-width apart.
● Slowly lower the bar towards your nipples.
● Press the bar back strongly to the start position.

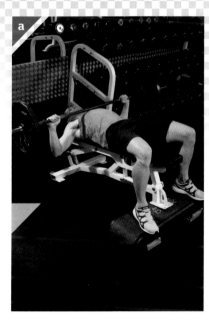
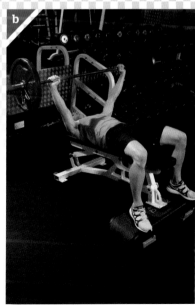

2a Incline dumbbell press

TARGETS
Chest, shoulders, triceps

WHY DO IT?
An incline bench places the focus on the upper part of your chest, as well as the front of your shoulders and triceps. The dumbbells allows for a greater range of motion.

HOW TO DO IT
● Lie on a bench set at a 30-45° angle holding a dumbbell in each hand at shoulder height.
● Keep your feet flat on the floor and your back against the bench.
● Press the weights directly above your head then slowly lower them again, flaring your elbows out to the side.

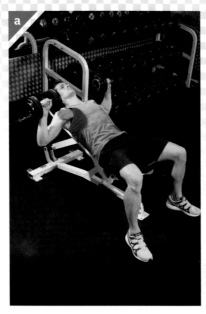
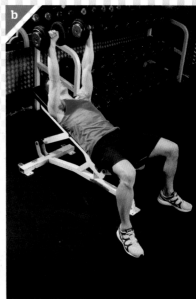

2b Cable crossover

TARGETS
Chest

WHY DO IT?
Using cables, rather than dumbbells, ensures that there is constant tension on your chest muscles throughout the move.

HOW TO DO IT
● Stand in the middle of a cable machine with a split stance holding a D-handle attachment in each hand, with the cable set above shoulder height.
● Keeping a natural arch in your back, your core braced and your upper body still, bring your hands down in an arc until they pass each other and your wrists are crossed.
● Pause and squeeze your pecs before returning to the start with a slow and controlled movement.

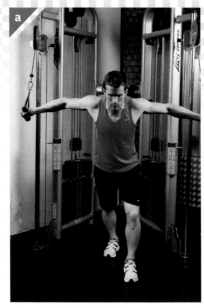
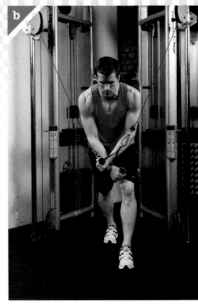

3a T press-up

TARGETS
Chest, triceps, shoulders, core

WHY DO IT?
This is a move that requires co-ordination and a strong core.

HOW TO DO IT
● Start in a press-up position, then lower your chest to the ground.
● Press back up then, at the top, lift one arm off the ground and point it up by twisting your torso.
● Return to the start and repeat with the other arm.

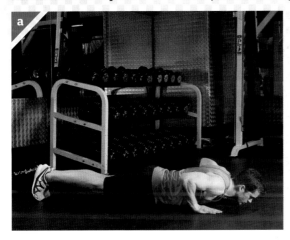

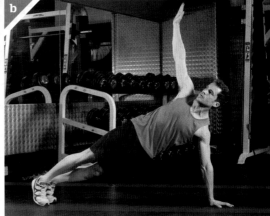

3b Plank

TARGETS
Core

WHY DO IT?
It works your core muscles to build a strong link between your upper and lower body.

HOW TO DO IT
● Hold your body in a straight line from head to heels with your elbows beneath your shoulders, keeping your feet together and your head looking down.
● Hold the position for as long as you can without letting your hips sag.

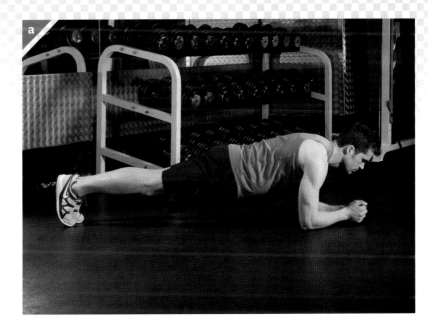

Workout three

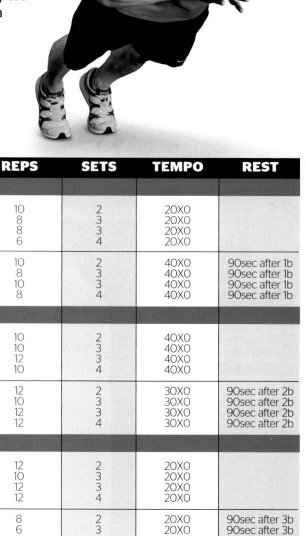

↘ This is another tough session that will not only work your chest but also your legs, arms, shoulders and core, as well as the small but important stabilising muscles that support your major joints. The workout ends with a plyometric bodyweight move – clap press-ups – to exhaust every last muscle fibre in your chest and build explosive power.

EXERCISE		WEEK	REPS	SETS	TEMPO	REST
SUPERSET 1						
1a Deadlift		1 2 3 4	10 8 8 6	2 3 3 4	20X0 20X0 20X0 20X0	
1b Incline bench press		1 2 3 4	10 8 10 8	2 3 3 4	40X0 40X0 40X0 40X0	90sec after 1b 90sec after 1b 90sec after 1b 90sec after 1b
SUPERSET 2						
2a Triceps dip		1 2 3 4	10 10 12 10	2 3 3 4	40X0 40X0 40X0 40X0	
2b Cable flye		1 2 3 4	12 10 12 12	2 3 3 4	30X0 30X0 30X0 30X0	90sec after 2b 90sec after 2b 90sec after 2b 90sec after 2b
SUPERSET 3						
3a Alternating dumbbell floor press		1 2 3 4	12 10 12 12	2 3 3 4	20X0 20X0 20X0 20X0	
3b Clap press-up		1 2 3 4	8 6 8 8	2 3 3 4	20X0 20X0 20X0 20X0	90sec after 3b 90sec after 3b 90sec after 3b 90sec after 3b

1a Deadlift

TARGETS
Total body

WHY DO IT?
This total-body move is a great way to start any session, firing up your muscles to set you on your muscle-building path.

HOW TO DO IT
- Grip the bar just outside your knees with your core braced, your shoulders retracted and over the bar and your back flat.
- Use your glutes to power the initial lift, pushing down through your heels.
- Keep the bar close to your body and, as it passes your knees, push your hips forwards. Keep your shoulders back throughout the move.

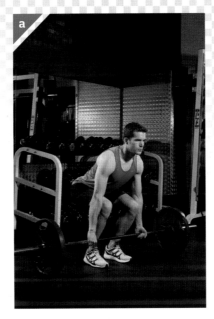
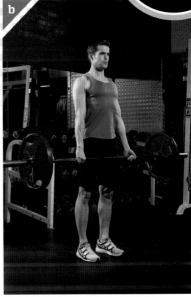

1b Incline bench press

TARGETS
Chest, shoulders, triceps

WHY DO IT?
Tilting the bench upwards places the focus on the upper part of your chest, as well as the front of your shoulders and triceps.

HOW TO DO IT
- Lie on a bench set at a 30-45˚ angle, holding a barbell with an overhand grip.
- Keep your feet flat on the floor and back against the bench.
- Slowly lower the weight to your chest, flaring your elbows out to the side, then press the weight directly above your head without locking out your elbows at the top.

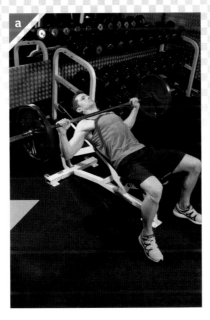
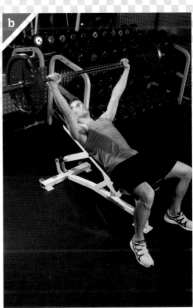

2a Triceps dip

TARGETS
Triceps, lower chest, shoulders

WHY DO IT?
The dip is one of the best moves to target all three parts of the triceps, as well as being great for working the lower chest, shoulders and your core, which must stay tight to prevent your legs swinging.

HOW TO DO IT
● Grip parallel bars, keeping your body upright.
● With your elbows pointing straight back, lower your body as far as you can comfortably go without stressing your shoulders.
● Keep your core braced and don't swing your legs for momentum.

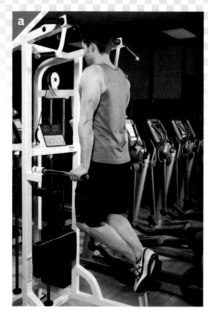
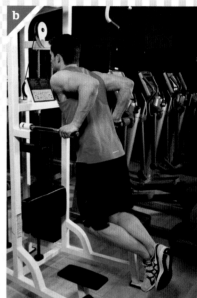

2b Cable flye

TARGETS
Chest

WHY DO IT?
It works your chest muscles through a full range of motion.

HOW TO DO IT
● Stand in the middle of a cable machine with a split stance holding a D-handle attachment in each hand, with the cable set above shoulder height.
● Keeping a natural arch in your back, your core braced and your upper body still, bring your hands down in an arc until they almost meet in front of your chest.
● Pause and squeeze your pecs before returning to the start with a slow and controlled movement.

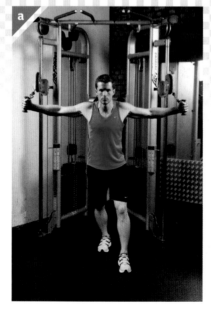
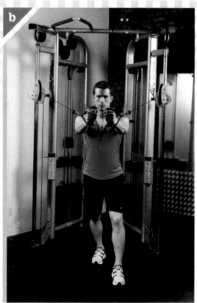

3a Alternating dumbbell floor press

TARGETS
Chest, triceps

WHY DO IT?
Alternating each arm works them independently for balanced gains, while using the floor rather than a bench improves stability.

HOW TO DO IT
● Lie flat on the floor with knees bent, holding a dumbbell in each hand with arms fully extended and pointing up.
● Lower one weight by bending at the elbow until your upper arm is horizontal, then press back up. Repeat with the other arm.

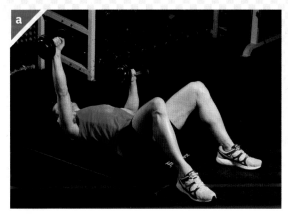
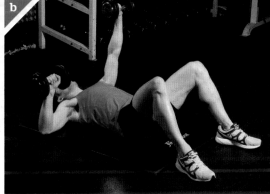

3b Clap press-up

TARGETS
Chest, triceps, shoulders, core

WHY DO IT?
Having to clap between press-ups means you have to push up from the floor very quickly, turning this exercise into an explosive muscle-building move.

HOW TO DO IT
● Start in a press-up position and lower your chest to the ground, keeping your elbows close to your sides.
● Press back up powerfully so that your hands leave the floor. Quickly clap them together.
● Land and descend into the next rep.

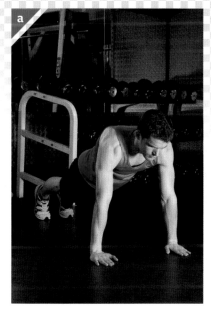
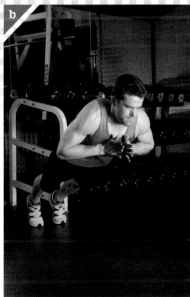

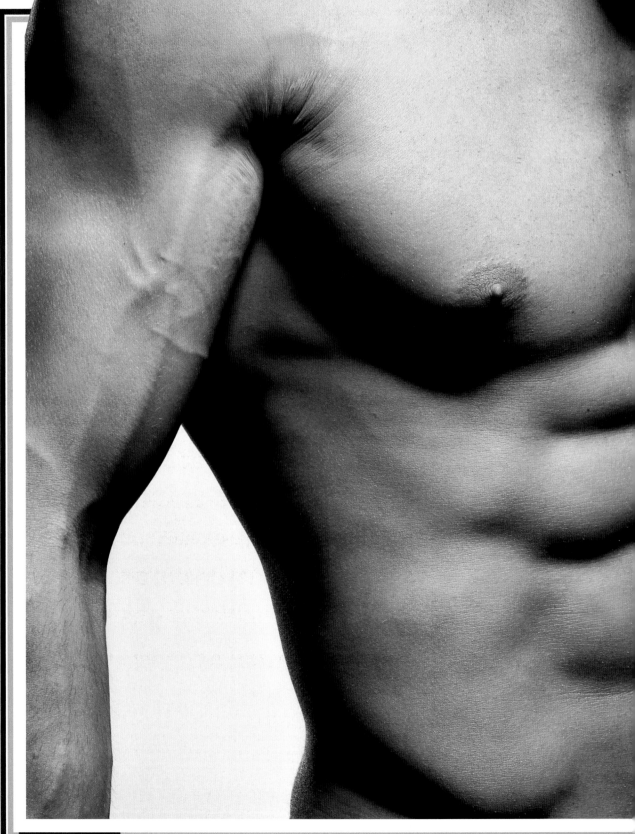

Get rock hard abs

Sculpt a solid six-pack with these abs-focused workouts

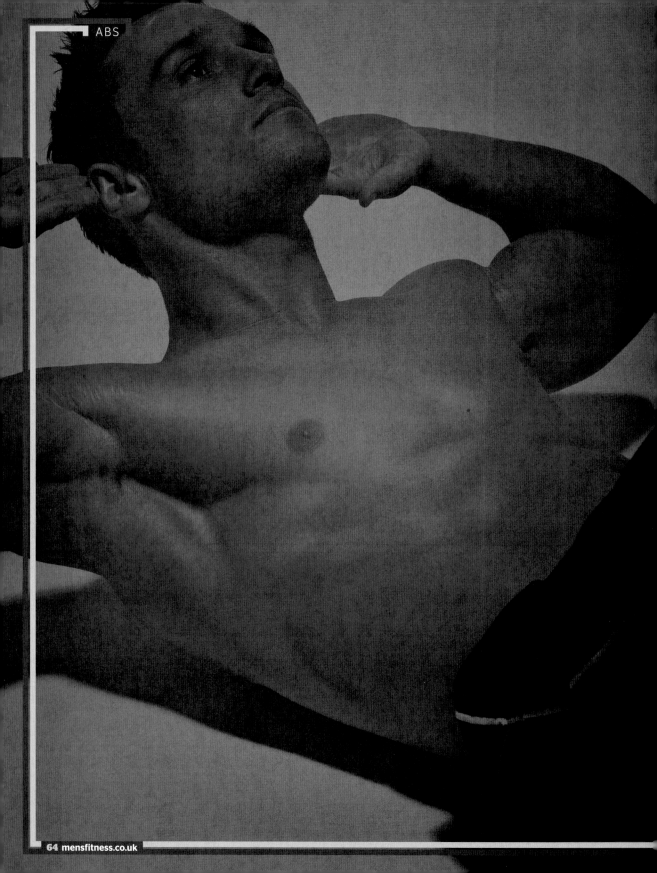

Abs of steel

COVER MODEL BODY

When you think of a *Men's Fitness* cover model, the first thing that comes to mind is a solid six-pack. But our models don't do many sit-ups. Building hard abs means making them work to stabilise your torso during heavy lifts, such as squats, and those that involve lifting a weight above your head, such as the shoulder press.

How to do the workouts

Make gains fast with these four muscle-specific training plans

There are four workouts in this chapter. Each of these programmes is based on doing three sessions per week for a total of four weeks.

The first plan is a foundation workout designed for men of all athletic abilities, so make sure you start off by following this one rather than jumping straight into one of the three main workouts.

For those of you new to this type of exercise it will build a solid base from which you can launch into the more intense workouts. And even if you are a more experienced trainer, there's still much to gain from starting with the basics. It will help correct any muscular imbalances you may have, allow you to correct any poor form habits you may have picked up and let you master some simple movement patterns, including bodyweight moves, that you may have neglected during most of your previous training regimes.

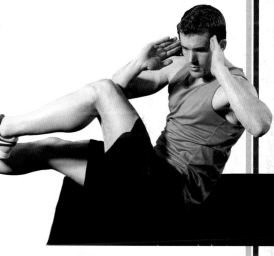

ANATOMY OF THE MUSCLE GROUP ABS

Your abs stabilise your trunk; they're responsible for forward and rotational movements; and they control side bending and back extension. Here's how.

❶ Transversus abdominis

This a deep-lying muscle that runs across your torso from side to side, holding your ribs in place and stabilising your pelvic area.

❷ Internal obliques

On top of the transversus abdominis lie your internal obliques. These run upwards from your hip, allowing you to bend and rotate to the sides.

❸ External obliques

The external obliques lie above the internal obliques, running in the opposite direction. They work alongside others to bend and rotate your torso.

❹ Rectus abdominis

This sheet of muscle is separated into segments, giving you the classic six-pack look when it is developed.

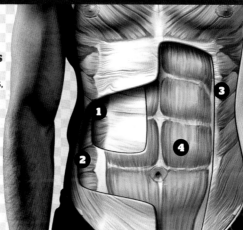

Foundation workout

This bodyweight workout begins with an explosive superset to increase your heart rate and prepare your muscles for the rest of the session. The final four abs-specific moves will begin to carve out your new six-pack while also building a solid, stable core.

EXERCISE		WEEK	REPS	SETS	TEMPO	REST
SUPERSET 1						
1a Tuck jump		1	8	2	X	
		2	10	2	X	
		3	8	3	X	
		4	10	3	X	
1b Press-up burpee		1	8	2	X	90sec after 1b
		2	10	2	X	90sec after 1b
		3	8	3	X	90sec after 1b
		4	10	3	X	90sec after 1b
SUPERSET 2						
2a Crunch		1	12	2	2020	
		2	15	2	2020	
		3	12	3	2020	
		4	15	3	2020	
2b Plank		1	1	2	10sec	90sec after 2b
		2	1	2	15sec	90sec after 2b
		3	1	3	15sec	90sec after 2b
		4	1	3	30sec	90sec after 2b
SUPERSET 3						
3a Two-point box		1	12	2	2010	
		2	15	2	2010	
		3	12	3	2010	
		4	15	3	2010	
3b Russian twist		1	8	2	2020	90sec after 3b
		2	10	2	2020	90sec after 3b
		3	8	3	2020	90sec after 3b
		4	10	3	2020	90sec after 3b

1a Tuck jump

TARGETS
Total body

WHY DO IT?
Fire up your heart rate and get your muscles warm with this plyometric bodyweight move.

HOW TO DO IT
- Stand tall with your feet closer than hip-width apart.
- Bend your knees, then jump up, tucking your knees up in front of you.
- Land and repeat.

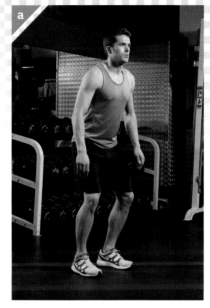

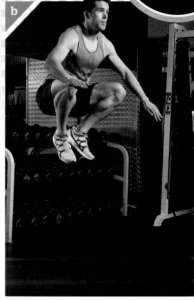

1b Press-up burpee

TARGETS
Total body

WHY DO IT?
This is a great move for working multiple muscle groups at once.

HOW TO DO IT
- Stand tall with your arms by your sides, then lower into a squat.
- As you reach the bottom of the squat, put your hands on the ground and kick your legs back until you are in a press-up position.
- Do a press-up, then bring your legs back underneath you and jump up.

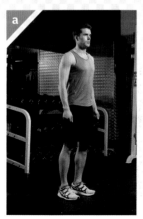

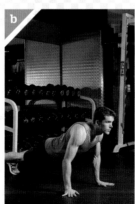

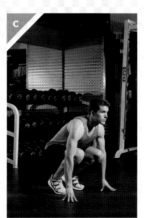

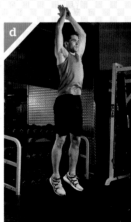

2a Crunch

TARGETS
Upper abs

WHY DO IT?
The classic move for targeting your upper abs – and still one of the best.

HOW TO DO IT
● Lie with your back flat on a mat with knees bent at 90˚, feet flat on the floor and fingers by your temples.
● Contract your abs to curl your chest towards your knees. Pause at the top of the move and squeeze your abs, then lower slowly to the start.

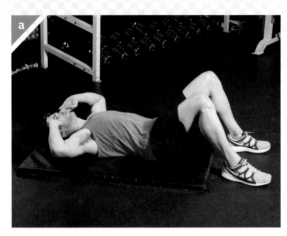
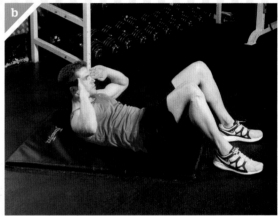

2b Plank

TARGETS
Core

WHY DO IT?
It works those deep-lying core muscles and builds a strong link between your upper and lower body.

HOW TO DO IT
● Hold your body in a straight line from head to heels with your elbows beneath your shoulders, feet together and head looking down.
● Hold the position for as long as you can without letting your hips sag.

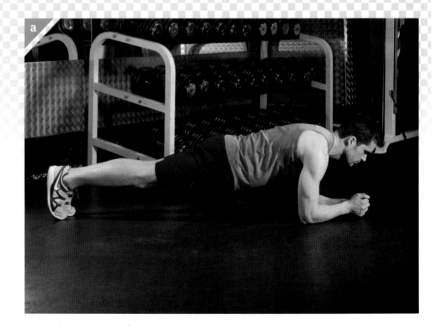

3a Two-point box

TARGETS
Core, lower back

WHY DO IT?
This moves works your deep core and lower-back muscles that are often neglected.

HOW TO DO IT
- Start on your hands and knees.
- Bring your left arm and right knee towards your stomach until they touch, then straighten them.
- Return to the start and repeat with the opposite arm and leg.

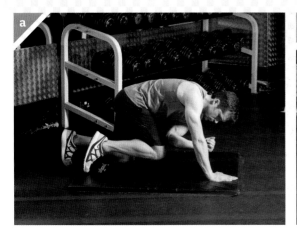
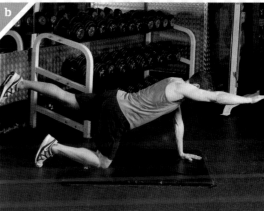

3b Russian twist

TARGETS
Lower abs, obliques

WHY DO IT?
This tough move keeps the focus on your lower abs and obliques while also working your core.

HOW TO DO IT
- Lie flat on your back with arms out to the sides and legs straight up in the air. Keep your shoulders and upper back on the mat throughout.
- Twist over to one side, keeping your legs straight. Go as far as you can to the side without letting your feet hit the floor. Reverse the move to the start and twist the other way.

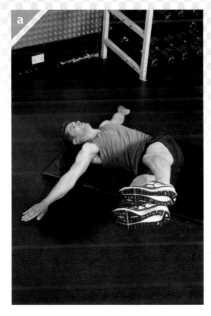
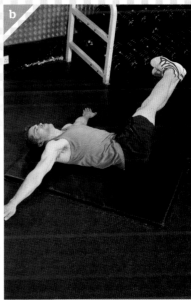

Workout one

Every single standing-up move works your core, which is why this session kicks off with a superset that will really test your midsection, as well as your legs, glutes, back and shoulders. You'll then target your abs from a variety of angles to fully fatigue your core before getting some well-earned rest.

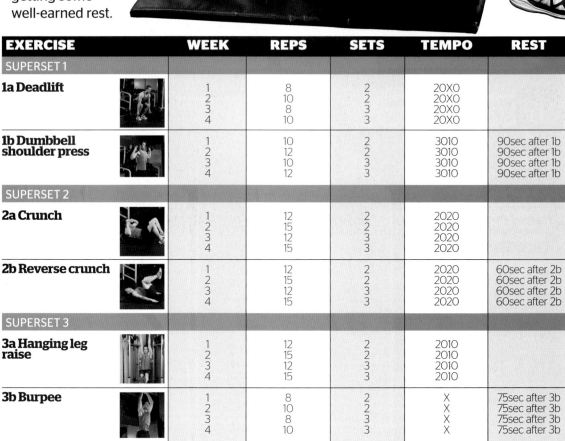

EXERCISE		WEEK	REPS	SETS	TEMPO	REST
SUPERSET 1						
1a Deadlift		1 2 3 4	8 10 8 10	2 2 3 3	20X0 20X0 20X0 20X0	
1b Dumbbell shoulder press		1 2 3 4	10 12 10 12	2 2 3 3	3010 3010 3010 3010	90sec after 1b 90sec after 1b 90sec after 1b 90sec after 1b
SUPERSET 2						
2a Crunch		1 2 3 4	12 15 12 15	2 2 3 3	2020 2020 2020 2020	
2b Reverse crunch		1 2 3 4	12 15 12 15	2 2 3 3	2020 2020 2020 2020	60sec after 2b 60sec after 2b 60sec after 2b 60sec after 2b
SUPERSET 3						
3a Hanging leg raise		1 2 3 4	12 15 12 15	2 2 3 3	2010 2010 2010 2010	
3b Burpee		1 2 3 4	8 10 8 10	2 2 3 3	X X X X	75sec after 3b 75sec after 3b 75sec after 3b 75sec after 3b

1a Deadlift

TARGETS
Total body

WHY DO IT?
The deadlift is an important move because so many muscle groups are involved, specifically the legs, glutes, back and the core, which must work hard to keep you stable.

HOW TO DO IT
● Grip the bar just outside your knees with your core braced, your shoulders retracted and over the bar and your back flat.
● Use your glutes to power the initial lift, pushing down through your heels.
● As the bar passes your knees, push your hips forward. Keep your shoulders back throughout the move.

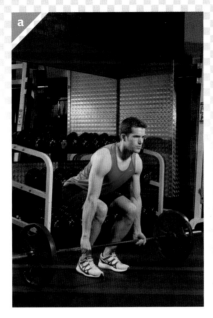
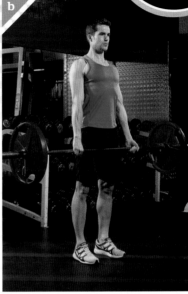

1b Dumbbell shoulder press

TARGETS
Shoulders, triceps, core

WHY DO IT?
This works your shoulders and triceps and performing it standing up means your core must be fully engaged to keep your torso stable.

HOW TO DO IT
● With your feet shoulder-width apart, hold a dumbbell in each hand at shoulder height.
● Keep your chest upright and your core muscles braced.
● Press the weights directly upwards, keeping your core braced, until your arms are extended overhead.
● Lower the weights again and repeat.

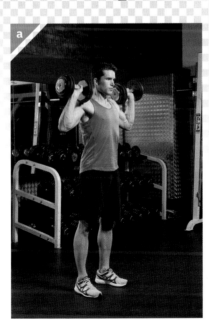
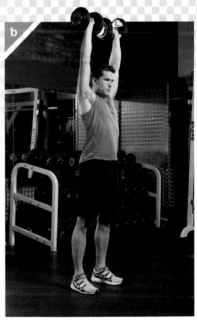

2a Crunch

TARGETS
Upper abs

WHY DO IT?
The classic move for targeting your upper abs – and still one of the best.

HOW TO DO IT
● Lie with your back flat on a mat with knees bent at 90˚, feet flat on the floor and fingers by your temples.
● Contract your abs to curl your chest towards your knees. Pause at the top of the move and squeeze your abs, then lower slowly to the start.

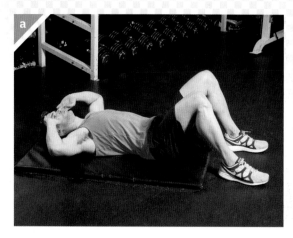
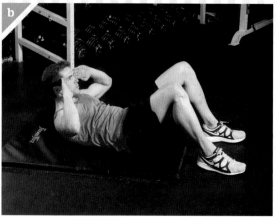

2b Reverse crunch

TARGETS
Lower abs

WHY DO IT?
It places the emphasis on your lower abs by hitting them from a new angle.

HOW TO DO IT
● Start with your back flat on the mat with your arms down by your sides, knees bent at 90˚ and feet flat.
● Contract your abs to lift your hips off the mat, then curl your knees towards your chest. Pause at the top, squeezing your abs, then lower back to the start.

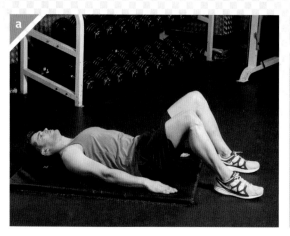
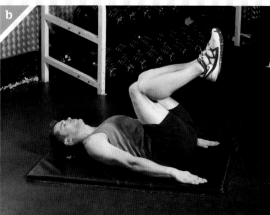

3a Hanging leg raise

TARGETS
Lower abs

WHY DO IT?
Keeping your legs straight while
you raise them forces your lower
abs to control the entire range of
motion. Lower your legs slowly
to work them even harder.

HOW TO DO IT
● Hang from a bar with
your body straight.
● Keeping your legs straight,
use your lower abs to raise
them up until they are
parallel with the ground, then
return slowly to the start.

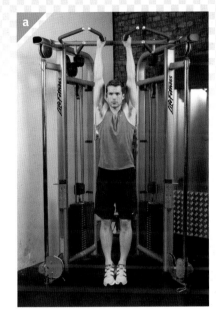
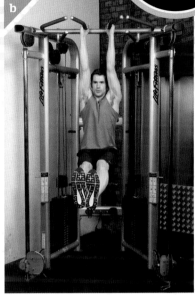

3b Burpee

TARGETS
Total body

WHY DO IT?
This works most major
muscle groups as well as
getting your heart rate high.

HOW TO DO IT
● Stand with your arms
by your sides, then
lower into a squat.
● As you reach the bottom
of the squat, put your hands
on the ground and kick
your legs back until you
are in a press-up position.
● Bring your legs back
underneath you, then
jump up off the ground.

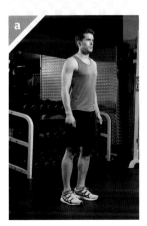
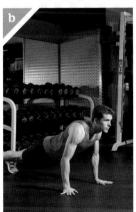
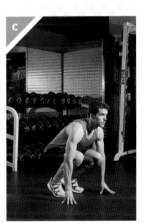
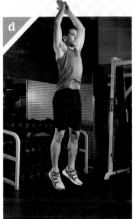

Workout two

Your core must work hard in the first superset to stabilise your torso through the duration of every rep. And it won't ease up after that with four tough abs-focused moves that work your entire core region from multiple angles to start sculpting a solid six-pack.

EXERCISE		WEEK	REPS	SETS	TEMPO	REST
SUPERSET 1						
1a Shoulder press		1	8	2	2010	
		2	8	3	2010	
		3	10	3	2010	
		4	12	3	2010	
1b Barbell lunge		1	10	2	20X0	90sec after 1b
		2	8	3	20X0	90sec after 1b
		3	10	3	20X0	90sec after 1b
		4	12	3	20X0	90sec after 1b
SUPERSET 2						
2a Barbell roll-out		1	8	2	2111	
		2	8	3	2111	
		3	10	3	2111	
		4	12	3	2111	
2b Medicine ball knee raise		1	12	2	2111	60sec after 2b
		2	15	3	2111	60sec after 2b
		3	15	3	2111	60sec after 2b
		4	20	3	2111	60sec after 2b
SUPERSET 3						
3a Plank		1	1	2	20sec	
		2	1	3	20sec	
		3	1	3	30sec	
		4	1	3	45sec	
3b Jackknife		1	12	2	2020	60sec after 2b
		2	12	3	2020	60sec after 2b
		3	15	3	2020	60sec after 2b
		4	15	3	2020	60sec after 2b

1a Shoulder press

TARGETS
Shoulders, triceps, core

WHY DO IT?
It mainly works the front and middle deltoids – two of the three major muscles that make up your shoulders – but also works your core, which must be fully engaged to keep you stable.

HOW TO DO IT
● Position a bar on your upper chest, gripping it with hands just wider than shoulder-width apart.
● Keep your chest upright and your core muscles braced.
● Press the bar directly upwards until your arms are straight.
● Lower the bar back to your chest slowly.

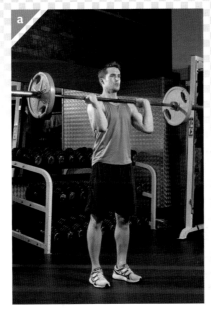
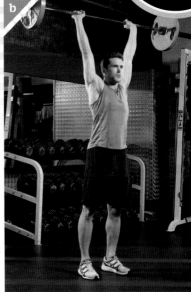

1b Barbell lunge

TARGETS
Quads, hams, glutes, core

WHY DO IT?
Lunges work the powerhouse lower-body muscles and many other stabilising muscles, including your core.

HOW TO DO IT
● Stand tall with a barbell resting on the back of your shoulders.
● Point your elbows behind you to retract your shoulder blades and keep your back upright and core braced throughout.
● Take a big step forward but keep your knee over your front foot – don't let it go beyond it. Lower until both knees are bent at 90˚, then push back off your front foot to return to the start position.

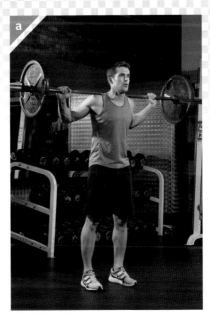
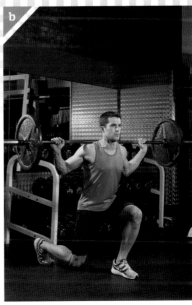

2a Barbell roll-out

TARGETS
Core

WHY DO IT?
This is a surprisingly tough move that works the entire abdominal region to carve a solid six-pack.

HOW TO DO IT
● Get on your knees with your arms in front holding the bar of a barbell.
● Roll forward, extending your abs, before rolling back to the start position.

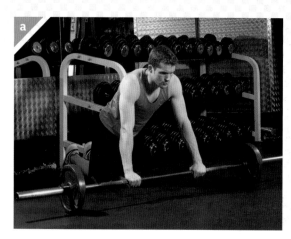
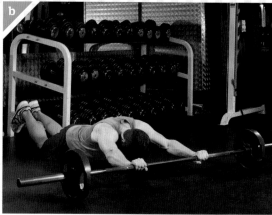

2b Medicine ball knee raise

TARGETS
Lower abs and core

WHY DO IT?
The additional weight of the ball forces your lower abs to work hard to raise your knees, while your core works to stabilise your upper body.

HOW TO DO IT
● Hang from a pull-up bar with a medicine ball held securely between your knees.
● Bend your knees and use your lower abs to draw them up towards your chest.
● Once your thighs are parallel to the floor, pause and then slowly return to the start.

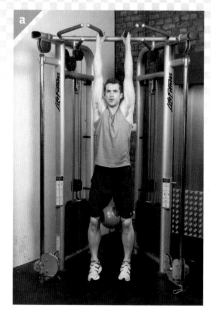
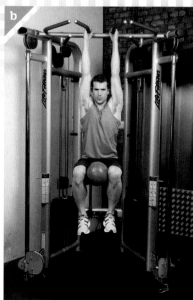

3a Plank

TARGETS
Core

WHY DO IT?
Nothing works your entire abdominal region as hard in such a short amount of time as the plank, the classic stability move. Every muscle must work together to keep your torso stable and prevent your hips from sagging.

HOW TO DO IT
● Hold your body in a straight line from head to heels with your elbows beneath your shoulders, feet together and head looking down.
● Hold the position for as long as you can without letting your hips sag.

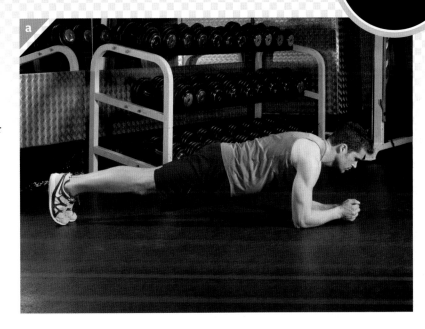

3b Jackknife

TARGETS
Abs

WHY DO IT?
Hit your upper and lower abs with this move that requires flexibility.

HOW TO DO IT
● Lie flat on your back with arms behind your head, off the floor, and feet together, also off the floor.
● Contract your abs to bring your hands and feet up over your stomach. Keep your legs straight. Return to the start.

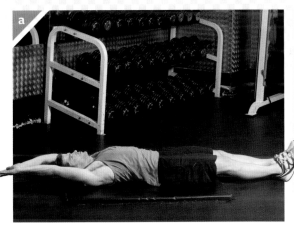

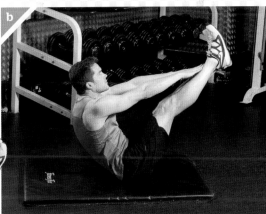

Workout three

This final workout builds on the first two by taxing your core by making it stabilise your torso during a tough first superset that targets all the major muscles of your upper and lower body. You'll then hit your abs and the deep-lying core muscles with four of the toughest bodyweight moves you can do.

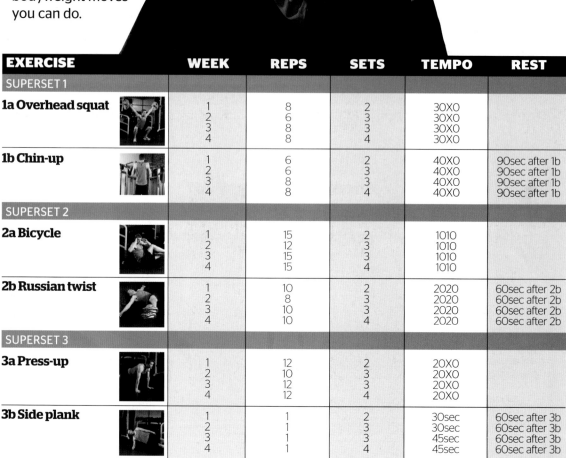

EXERCISE		WEEK	REPS	SETS	TEMPO	REST
SUPERSET 1						
1a Overhead squat		1	8	2	30X0	
		2	6	3	30X0	
		3	8	3	30X0	
		4	8	4	30X0	
1b Chin-up		1	6	2	40X0	90sec after 1b
		2	6	3	40X0	90sec after 1b
		3	8	3	40X0	90sec after 1b
		4	8	4	40X0	90sec after 1b
SUPERSET 2						
2a Bicycle		1	15	2	1010	
		2	12	3	1010	
		3	15	3	1010	
		4	15	4	1010	
2b Russian twist		1	10	2	2020	60sec after 2b
		2	8	3	2020	60sec after 2b
		3	10	3	2020	60sec after 2b
		4	10	4	2020	60sec after 2b
SUPERSET 3						
3a Press-up		1	12	2	20X0	
		2	10	3	20X0	
		3	12	3	20X0	
		4	12	4	20X0	
3b Side plank		1	1	2	30sec	60sec after 3b
		2	1	3	30sec	60sec after 3b
		3	1	3	45sec	60sec after 3b
		4	1	4	45sec	60sec after 3b

1a Overhead squat

TARGETS
Quads, hams, glutes, core

WHY DO IT?
This tough twist on the classic squat is the final part of the snatch Olympic lift. It will test your posture, core strength and shoulder mobility to the max, but getting better at this will benefit a host of other moves.

HOW TO DO IT
● Stand tall holding a barbell overhead with a wide grip.
● Your feet should be shoulder-width apart, your core braced, with a natural arch in your back.
● Squat down as low as you can without allowing your back to arch.
● Drive back up through your heels to complete the move.

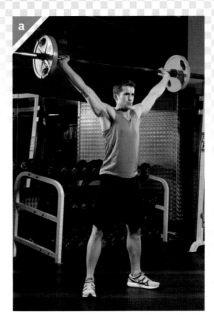
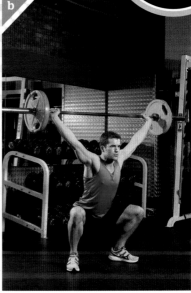

1b Chin-up

TARGETS
Biceps, upper back, core

WHY DO IT?
Using an underhand grip shifts the focus to your biceps, making the move slightly easier while still taxing all the major muscles of your upper back.

HOW TO DO IT
● Grab the bars with an underhand grip. If using a straight bar your hands should be shoulder-width apart.
● Start from a dead hang with your arms fully extended.
● Pull yourself up by squeezing your lats together.
● Once your chin is higher than your hands, pause briefly, then slowly lower back to the start.

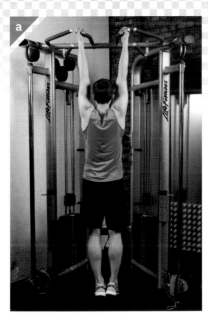
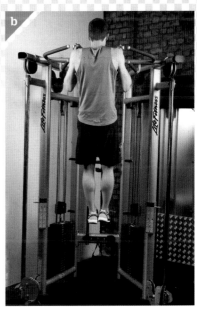

2a Bicycle

TARGETS
Abs, obliques

WHY DO IT?
Another timeless abs move. Do it quickly but in a controlled manner to exhaust the your muscle fibres.

HOW TO DO IT
● Lie flat on your back. Crunch up and bring your right elbow to meet your left knee, then return to the start.
● Repeat, alternating sides.

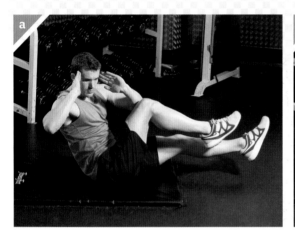
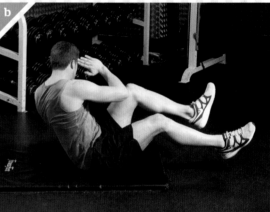

2b Russian twist

TARGETS
Lower abs, obliques

WHY DO IT?
Keep the focus on your lower abs and obliques with another advanced move that requires a stable core.

HOW TO DO IT
● Lie flat on your back with arms out to the sides and legs straight up in the air. Keep your shoulders and upper back on the mat throughout.
● Twist over to one side, keeping your legs straight. Go as far as you can to the side without letting your feet hit the floor. Reverse the move to the start and twist the other way.

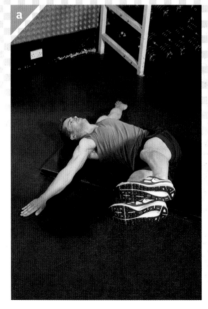
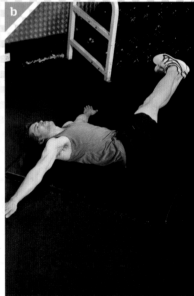

3a Press-up

TARGETS
Chest, triceps

WHY DO IT?
Press-ups require your chest, shoulder, triceps and core muscles to work hard to lower, then lift, your torso.

HOW TO DO IT
● Start with your hands shoulder-width apart and body straight.
● Lower yourself until your elbows reach 90°, then press back up.

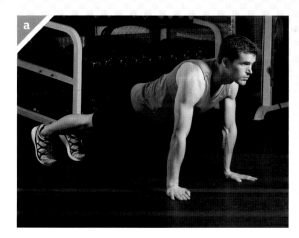
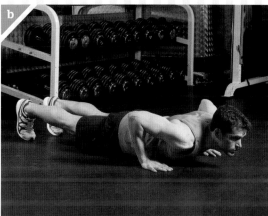

3b Side plank

TARGETS
Core, obliques

WHY DO IT?
Holding your body straight will build a powerful core to improve your posture.

HOW TO DO IT
● With your elbow directly underneath your shoulder, hold your body in a straight line from head to feet.
● Hold the position for as long as you can without letting your hips sag, then repeat on the other side.

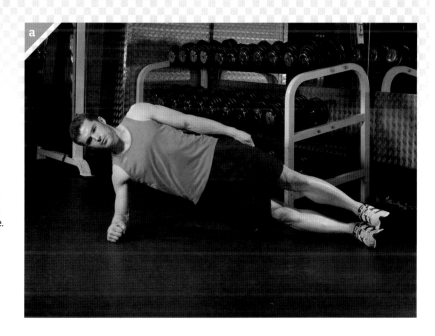

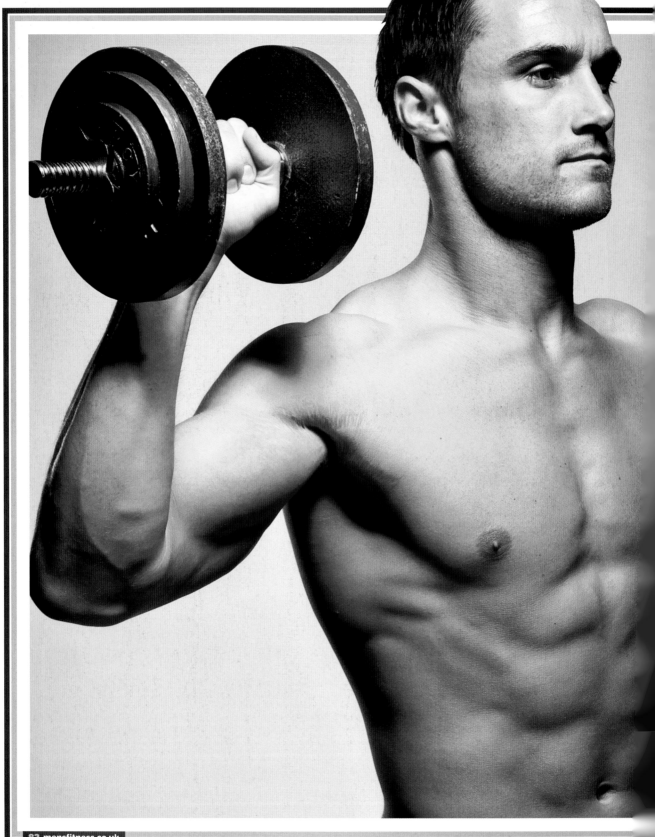

Build broad shoulders

Create a wide, V-shaped torso
by getting boulder shoulders

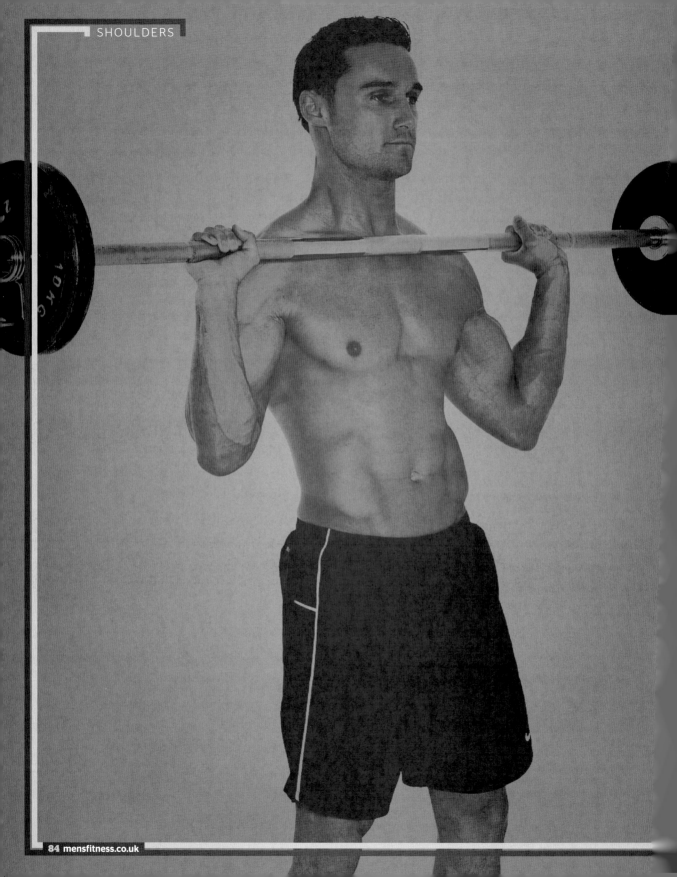

Boulder shoulders

One thing that defines *Men's Fitness* magazine cover models is their V-shaped torso. Wide, broad shoulders not only look good in themselves, they also make you look slimmer at the waist, even if you are carrying a little excess weight. But building big shoulders requires careful planning, because the shoulder joint is one of the most complicated joints in your body. Here's how to do it.

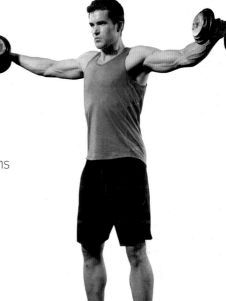

How to do the workouts
Make gains fast with these four muscle-specific training plans

There are four workouts in this chapter. Each of these programmes is based on doing three sessions per week for a total of four weeks.

The first plan is a foundation workout designed for men of all athletic abilities, so make sure you start off by following this one rather than jumping straight into one of the three main workouts.

For those of you new to this type of exercise it will build a solid base from which you can launch into the more intense workouts. And even if you are a more experienced trainer, there's still much to gain from starting with the basics. It will help correct any muscular imbalances you may have, allow you to correct any poor form habits you may have picked up and let you master some simple movement patterns, including bodyweight moves, that you may have neglected during most of your previous training regimes.

ANATOMY OF THE MUSCLE GROUP SHOULDERS

Deltoids

This three-part muscle goes around the shoulder joint. The anterior (front) deltoid starts on the collarbone, the medial (middle) deltoid starts on the top of the shoulder and the posterior (rear) deltoid starts on the shoulder blade. They all also join to the upper arm bone.

The anterior deltoid is involved in pushing moves that also work the chest, such as the bench press. The medial deltoid is responsible for lifting your arms straight overhead and the posterior deltoid is called on when you raise your arms out from your sides.

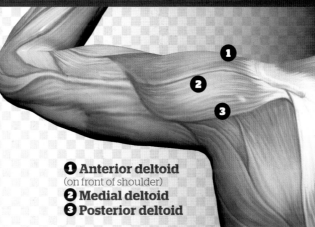

❶ Anterior deltoid
(on front of shoulder)
❷ Medial deltoid
❸ Posterior deltoid

Foundation workout

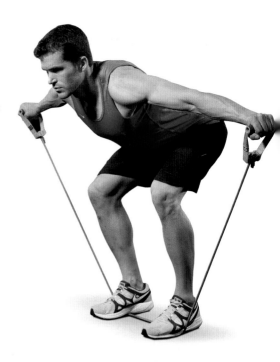

The shoulder joint is one of the most delicate in the human body because it's the most mobile, and its intricate design means you need to make it strong and stable before hitting it with any big lifts. This workout will do just that, as well as getting your heart pumping to burn fat.

EXERCISE		WEEK	REPS	SETS	TEMPO	REST
SUPERSET 1						
1a Tuck jump		1	10	2	X	
		2	12	2	X	
		3	10	3	X	
		4	12	3	X	
1b Bodyweight squat		1	12	2	3010	90sec after 1b
		2	15	2	3010	90sec after 1b
		3	12	3	3010	90sec after 1b
		4	15	3	3010	90sec after 1b
SUPERSET 2						
2a Inverted shoulder press		1	10	2	2010	
		2	12	2	2010	
		3	10	3	2010	
		4	12	3	2010	
2b Dumbbell shoulder press		1	10	2	2010	90sec after 2b
		2	12	2	2010	90sec after 2b
		3	10	3	2010	90sec after 2b
		4	12	3	2010	90sec after 2b
SUPERSET 3						
3a Stretch band lateral raise		1	12	2	2010	
		2	15	2	2010	
		3	12	3	2010	
		4	15	3	2010	
3b Dorsal raise with shoulder rotation		1	12	2	2010	90sec after 3b
		2	15	2	2010	90sec after 3b
		3	12	3	2010	90sec after 3b
		4	15	3	2010	90sec after 3b

1a Tuck jump

TARGETS
Total body

WHY DO IT?
Fire up your heart rate and get your muscles warm with this plyometric bodyweight move.

HOW TO DO IT
- Stand tall with feet closer than hip-width apart.
- Bend your knees, then jump up, tucking your knees up in front of you.
- Land and repeat.

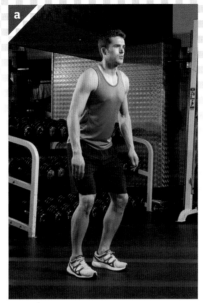
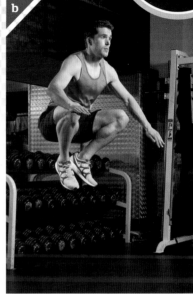

1b Bodyweight squat

TARGETS
Total body

WHY DO IT?
Mastering the correct form of a bodyweight squat means you'll make quicker progress when adding additional weight through a barbell or dumbbell. Hold your hands straight above you to activate the shoulder joint.

HOW TO DO IT
- Stand with your feet shoulder-width apart and pointing out slightly with your arms raised.
- Keeping your core braced and a natural arch in your back, squat down until your thighs are parallel to the floor, then push back up through your heels.

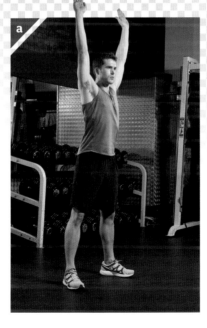
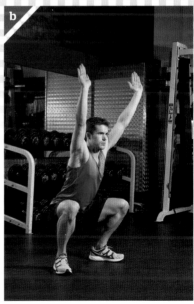

2a Inverted shoulder press

TARGETS
Shoulders, triceps, core

WHY DO IT?
The best way to work your shoulders without weights, this move also requires a strong core.

HOW TO DO IT
● Start with feet on a bench and your hands shoulder-width apart on the floor, so your body forms an inverted V-shape.

● Bend your elbows to slowly lower your body until your face almost touches the floor before pushing back up powerfully.

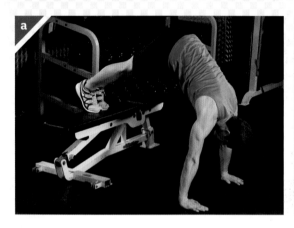

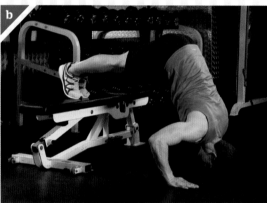

2b Dumbbell shoulder press

TARGETS
Shoulders, triceps

WHY DO IT?
This works your shoulders and triceps and performing it standing up means your core must be fully engaged to keep your torso stable.

HOW TO DO IT
● With your feet shoulder-width apart, hold a dumbbell in each hand at shoulder height.
● Keep your chest upright and your core muscles braced.
● Press the weights directly upwards, keeping your core braced, until your arms are extended overhead.
● Lower the weights again and repeat.

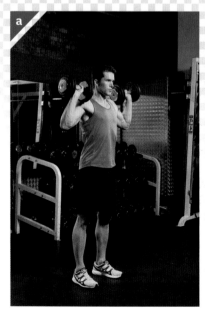

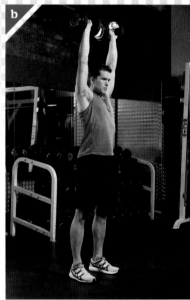

3a Stretch band lateral raise

TARGETS
Shoulders

WHY DO IT?
Using dumbbells for this move puts a lot of pressure on your delicate shoulder joint. The stretch band reduces this stress, allowing you to perfect the movement until you're ready to use a heavier weight.

HOW TO DO IT
● Hold a stretch band in each hand with the middle secured underfoot.
● Bend forward from the hips, keeping your arms by your sides.
● Keeping a slight bend in your elbows, slowly raise your arms as high as they can comfortably go.
● Slowly return to the start, controlling the tension in the band on the way down.

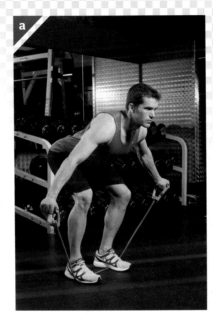
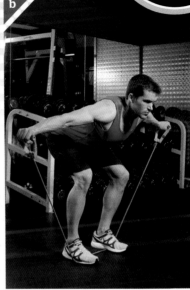

3b Dorsal raise with shoulder rotation

TARGETS
Rotator cuff, lower back

WHY DO IT?
As well as working your lower back, a weak spot for many men, this move also improves the strength of the delicate rotator cuff muscles that must be strong to allow you to lift heavier weights.

HOW TO DO IT
● Lie face-down on a mat with your arms straight out in front of you.
● As you raise your torso off the mat, rotate your arms round and out to the side, hold at the top, then return to the start.

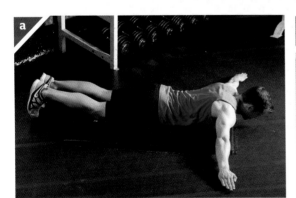
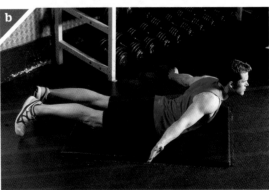

Workout one

This sessions starts with a superset designed both to warm up your shoulder joint fully and to hit it hard with the best big move for creating broad shoulders. The final supersets build upon this with isolation moves that target specific parts of the shoulders directly.

EXERCISE		WEEK	REPS	SETS	TEMPO	REST
SUPERSET 1						
1a Shoulder press		1	8	2	3010	
		2	10	2	3010	
		3	8	3	3010	
		4	10	3	3010	
1b Cuban press		1	10	2	3030	90sec after 1b
		2	12	2	3030	90sec after 1b
		3	10	3	3030	90sec after 1b
		4	12	3	3030	90sec after 1b
SUPERSET 2						
2a Dumbbell squat to curl to press		1	10	2	2020	
		2	12	2	2020	
		3	10	3	2020	
		4	12	3	2020	
2b Shrug		1	10	2	1211	90sec after 2b
		2	12	2	1211	90sec after 2b
		3	10	3	1211	90sec after 2b
		4	12	3	1211	90sec after 2b
SUPERSET 3						
3a Lateral raise		1	8	2	2010	
		2	10	2	2010	
		3	8	3	2010	
		4	10	3	2010	
3b Front raise		1	8	2	2010	90sec after 3b
		2	10	2	2010	90sec after 3b
		3	8	3	2010	90sec after 3b
		4	10	3	2010	90sec after 3b

1a Shoulder press

TARGETS
Shoulders, triceps, core

WHY DO IT?
The shoulder press is a hugely effective upper-body lift for adding size and strength to this major muscle group.

HOW TO DO IT
- With your feet shoulder-width apart, position a bar on your upper chest, gripping it with hands just wider than shoulder-width apart.
- Keep your chest upright and your core muscles braced.
- Press the bar directly upwards until your arms are extended overhead.
- Lower the bar back to your chest and repeat.

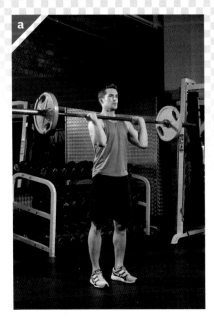
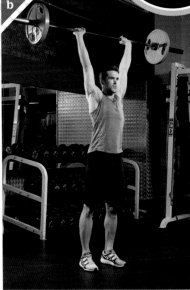

1b Barbell Cuban press

TARGETS
Shoulders

WHY DO IT?
It works the rotator cuff – the small but vital stabilising muscles of the shoulder joint. Use a light weight at first.

HOW TO DO IT
- Stand tall with your core braced, holding a barbell at the top of your thighs.
- Lift the bar by raising your arms out to the sides until your elbows are bent at 90°.
- Rotate your arms so your forearms point up, keeping your biceps horizontal.
- Press the bar directly overhead, then reverse the movement back down to the start.

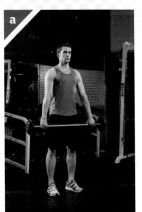
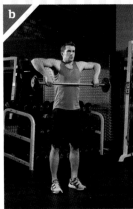
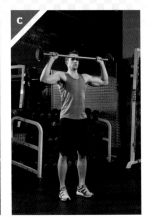
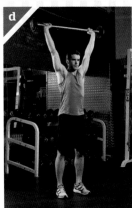

2a Dumbbell squat to curl to press

TARGETS
Total body

WHY DO IT?
It works most of your major muscle groups for a big growth-hormone response.

HOW TO DO IT
● Stand tall, holding a dumbbell in each hand, then squat down.
● Stand back up, curling the weights up, keeping your elbows close to your sides.
● From there, press the weights directly above your head. Reverse the entire movement back to the start.

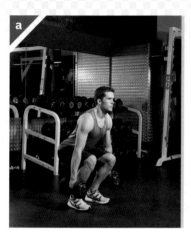
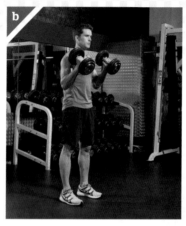
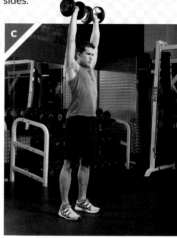

2b Shrug

TARGETS
Shoulders, traps

WHY DO IT?
Shrugs have a limited range of motion compared with most lifts. This means you can go really heavy on the weights to build big, strong traps and create wide shoulders.

HOW TO DO IT
● Stand between two heavy dumbbells, then squat down, grip the weights outside your hips and stand up, keeping your core braced.
● Shrug your shoulders up towards your ears, keeping your arms straight.
● Hold at the top before slowly lowering the weights again.

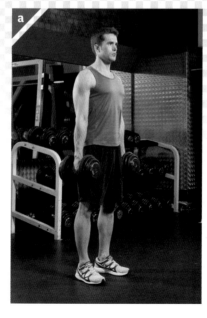
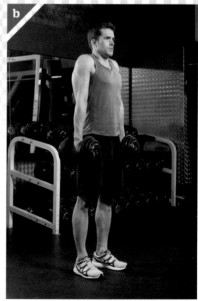

3a Lateral raise

TARGETS
Shoulders

WHY DO IT?
The lateral raise is one of the best moves for isolating the deltoids, especially those on the side of your upper arms. Keep the weights light and control the move from start to finish.

HOW TO DO IT
● Stand tall with core braced and feet apart, holding a light dumbbell in each hand by your sides with palms facing one another.
● Keeping a slight bend in your elbows, raise the weights out to the sides using your muscles and not momentum.
● Stop at shoulder height and pause for a second, then lower slowly.

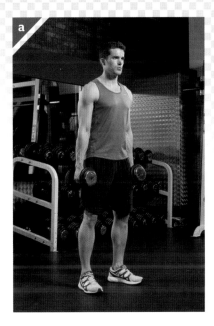
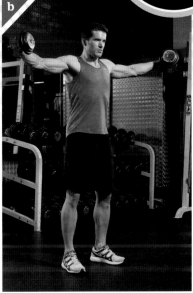

3b Front raise

TARGETS
Shoulders

WHY DO IT?
The front raise places greater emphasis on the front of your shoulders. As with the lateral raise, keep the weights light at first.

HOW TO DO IT
● Stand tall with core braced and feet apart, holding a light dumbbell in each hand by your sides with palms facing one another.
● Keeping a slight bend in your elbows, raise the weights out in front of you, using your muscles and not momentum.
● Stop at shoulder height, pause, then lower slowly.

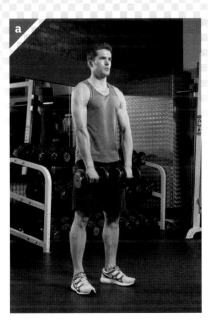
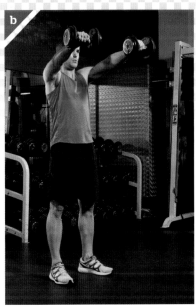

Workout two

We can't say this enough: it's crucial to start easy when training the shoulders, which is why this session begins with two of the best moves to train the rotator cuff, the tiny but invaluable muscles that are responsible for turning the shoulder joint. After this you'll blitz the shoulders, chest and triceps for rapid growth.

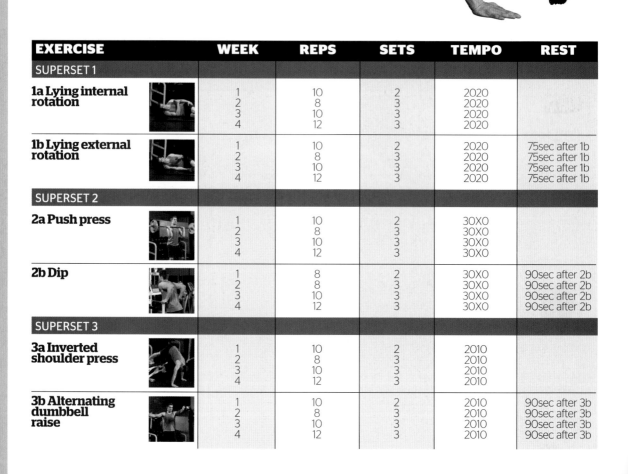

EXERCISE		WEEK	REPS	SETS	TEMPO	REST
SUPERSET 1						
1a Lying internal rotation		1 2 3 4	10 8 10 12	2 3 3 3	2020 2020 2020 2020	
1b Lying external rotation		1 2 3 4	10 8 10 12	2 3 3 3	2020 2020 2020 2020	75sec after 1b 75sec after 1b 75sec after 1b 75sec after 1b
SUPERSET 2						
2a Push press		1 2 3 4	10 8 10 12	2 3 3 3	30X0 30X0 30X0 30X0	
2b Dip		1 2 3 4	8 8 10 12	2 3 3 3	30X0 30X0 30X0 30X0	90sec after 2b 90sec after 2b 90sec after 2b 90sec after 2b
SUPERSET 3						
3a Inverted shoulder press		1 2 3 4	10 8 10 12	2 3 3 3	2010 2010 2010 2010	
3b Alternating dumbbell raise		1 2 3 4	10 8 10 12	2 3 3 3	2010 2010 2010 2010	90sec after 3b 90sec after 3b 90sec after 3b 90sec after 3b

1a Lying internal rotation

TARGETS
Rotator cuff

WHY DO IT?
To warm up those small but crucial stabilising muscles that support the shoulder joint. A strong rotator cuff will increase your ability in almost every upper-body lift.

HOW TO DO IT
● Lie on your side, holding a light dumbbell in the hand closest to the floor, with your elbow bent at 90˚.
● Keeping your elbow by your side, rotate your hand up until the weight is by your opposing upper arm, then slowly reverse back to the start.
● Repeat with your other arm.

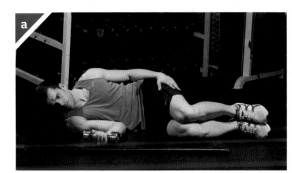
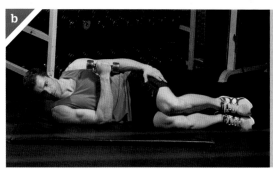

1b Lying external rotation

TARGETS
Rotator cuff

WHY DO IT?
This works the rotator cuff in the opposite direction to the first move to warm up the muscles thoroughly before the heavy lifting begins.

HOW TO DO IT
● Lie on your side, holding a light dumbbell in the hand furthest from the floor with your elbow bent at 90˚.
● Keeping your elbow on your side, rotate your hand up until your forearm is vertical, then slowly reverse back to the start.
● Repeat with your other arm.

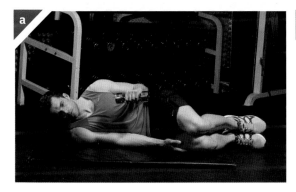
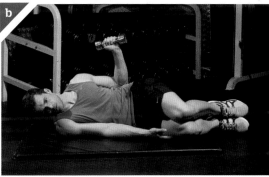

2a Push press

TARGETS
Legs, core, shoulders

WHY DO IT?
Using your legs to assist the move allows you to lift heavier, priming your muscles for growth.

HOW TO DO IT
● Stand with feet shoulder-width apart with the bar resting across the front of your shoulders.
● Bend your knees slightly then stand up straight to generate momentum. As you do, press the bar directly overhead.
● Slowly lower the weight back to the start position.

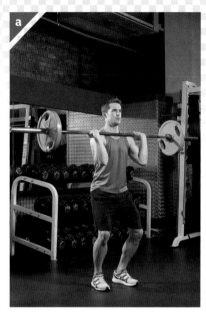
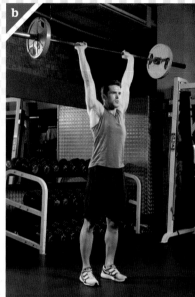

2b Triceps dip

TARGETS
Triceps, lower chest, shoulders

WHY DO IT?
As well as being one of the best moves for working the triceps, the dip hits the front shoulders hard.

HOW TO DO IT
● Grip parallel bars, keeping your body upright.
● With your elbows pointing straight back, lower your body as far as you can comfortably go without stressing your shoulders.
● Keep your core braced and don't swing your legs for momentum.

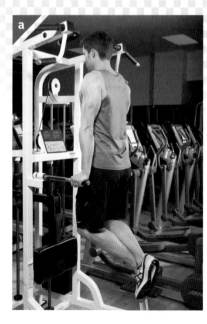
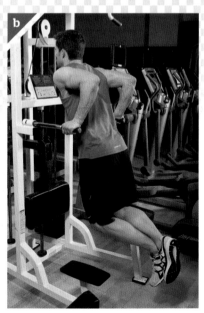

3a Inverted shoulder press

TARGETS
Shoulders, triceps

WHY DO IT?
It's simply the best way to work your shoulders without weights.

HOW TO DO IT
● Put your feet on a bench and your hands shoulder-width apart on the floor, so your body forms a V-shape.
● Bend your elbows to slowly lower your head almost to the floor, then push back up powerfully.

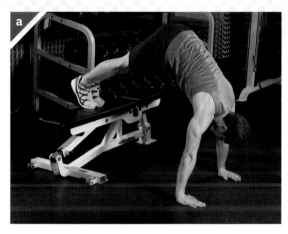
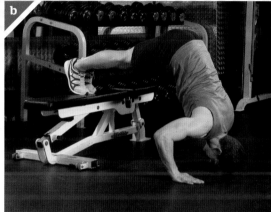

3b Alternating dumbbell raise

TARGETS
Shoulders

WHY DO IT?
Working each arm independently ensures balanced growth.

HOW TO DO IT
● Stand tall with a dumbbell in each hand at shoulder height.
● Lift one weight out to the side and one out to the front.
● Alternate arms with each rep.

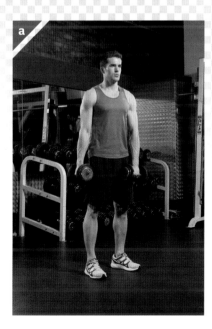
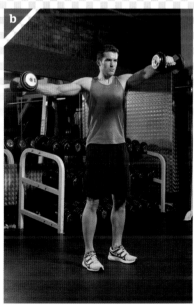

Workout three

The first superset of this session not only works two major muscle groups (shoulders and back) at the same time, it'll also get your heart rate soaring as it pumps blood from one end of your body to the other. You'll then hit the front and back of the shoulders, as well as your powerful traps to craft that V-shaped torso every man wants.

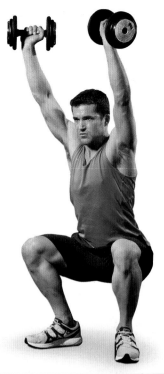

EXERCISE		WEEK	REPS	SETS	TEMPO	REST
SUPERSET 1						
1a Dumbbell lunge to press		1 2 3 4	10 10 12 10	2 3 3 4	2020 2020 2020 2020	
1b Back of steel		1 2 3 4	6 4 6 6	2 3 3 4	2121 2121 2121 2121	90sec after 1b 90sec after 1b 90sec after 1b 90sec after 1b
SUPERSET 2						
2a Arnold press		1 2 3 4	10 8 10 10	2 3 3 4	2020 2020 2020 2020	
2b Reverse dumbbell flye		1 2 3 4	10 8 10 10	2 3 3 4	2010 2010 2010 2010	90sec after 2b 90sec after 2b 75sec after 2b 75sec after 2b
SUPERSET 3						
3a Alternating wide dumbbell shoulder press		1 2 3 4	12 10 12 12	2 3 3 4	2010 2010 2010 2010	
3b Upright row		1 2 3 4	8 6 8 6	2 3 3 4	20X0 20X0 20X0 20X0	90sec after 3b 90sec after 3b 75sec after 3b 75sec after 3b

TARGETS
Legs, core, shoulders

WHY DO IT?
Work your legs, core and shoulders with this tough move that requires co-ordination and balance.

HOW TO DO IT
- Stand tall holding a dumbbell in each hand at shoulder height.
- Take a big step forward with one leg while pressing both weights directly above your head. Lunge until both knees are bent at 90˚.
- Push back off your front foot and lower the weights again, then repeat with the other leg.

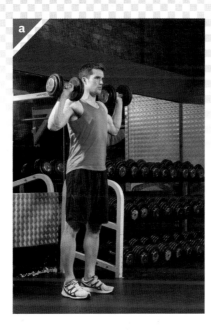
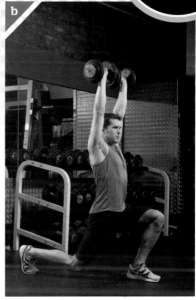

TARGETS
Legs, core, shoulders

WHY DO IT?
Not only does this move work your shoulders, it also really taxes your abs and legs to hold the squat position while lifting. Start with light dumbbells.

HOW TO DO IT
- Stand tall with a dumbbell in each hand with both arms directly above your head, then squat down, keeping your arms straight up.
- Squat until your thighs are parallel to the ground, then lower the weights down to shoulder height.
- Press the weights back up and continue with the press reps in a squatting position.

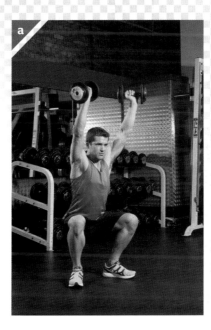
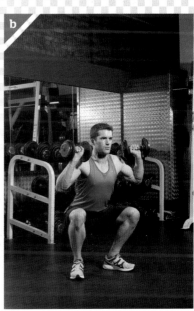

2a Arnold press

TARGETS
Shoulders, triceps

WHY DO IT?
This variation combines a pressing action with a rotational one to hit your deltoids from several angles.

HOW TO DO IT
● Sit on an upright bench holding a dumbbell in each hand with palms facing you.
● Keep your feet flat on the floor and back against the bench.
● Press the weights up, rotating your palms as you go so that you end the movement with arms directly overhead with your palms facing away.
● Reverse the action back down to the start.

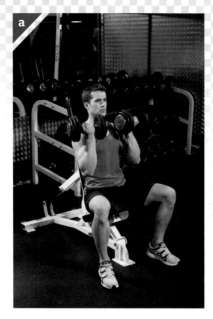
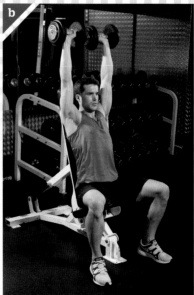

2b Reverse dumbbell flye

TARGETS
Rear deltoids

WHY DO IT?
This is a great move for targeting the muscle that makes up the rear part of your shoulders. It's often neglected in favour of working the other two muscles but you need balanced growth to ensure you get wide shoulders.

HOW TO DO IT
● Stand holding a dumbbell in each hand.
● Bend forward from the hips and, keeping a slight bend in your elbows, raise the weights out to your sides to shoulder height, the return to the start.

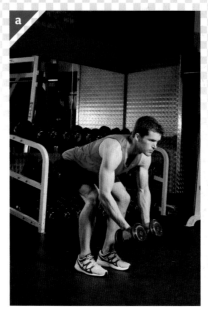
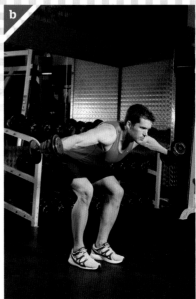

3a Alternating wide shoulder press

TARGETS
Shoulders

WHY DO IT?
A slight twist turns the humble shoulder press into this tough move that will build wide shoulders.

HOW TO DO IT
● Stand with feet hip-width apart with a dumbbell held in each hand at shoulder height.
● One hand at a time, press the dumb-bell up and out to the side at a 45˚ angle.
● Slowly return to the start and repeat with the other arm.

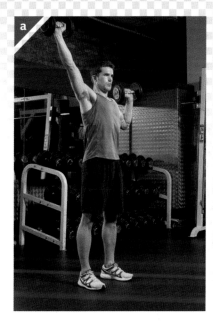
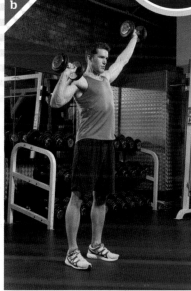

3b Upright row

TARGETS
Shoulders, traps

WHY DO IT?
This move mainly works your traps and shoulders to help craft a strong and wide torso.

HOW TO DO IT
● Stand tall holding a barbell with an overhand grip slightly narrower than shoulder width.
● Shrug the bar up towards your chin, leading with your elbows.
● Slowly lower the bar back to the start.

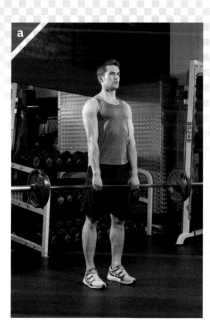
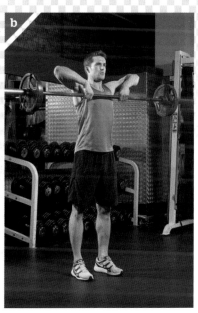

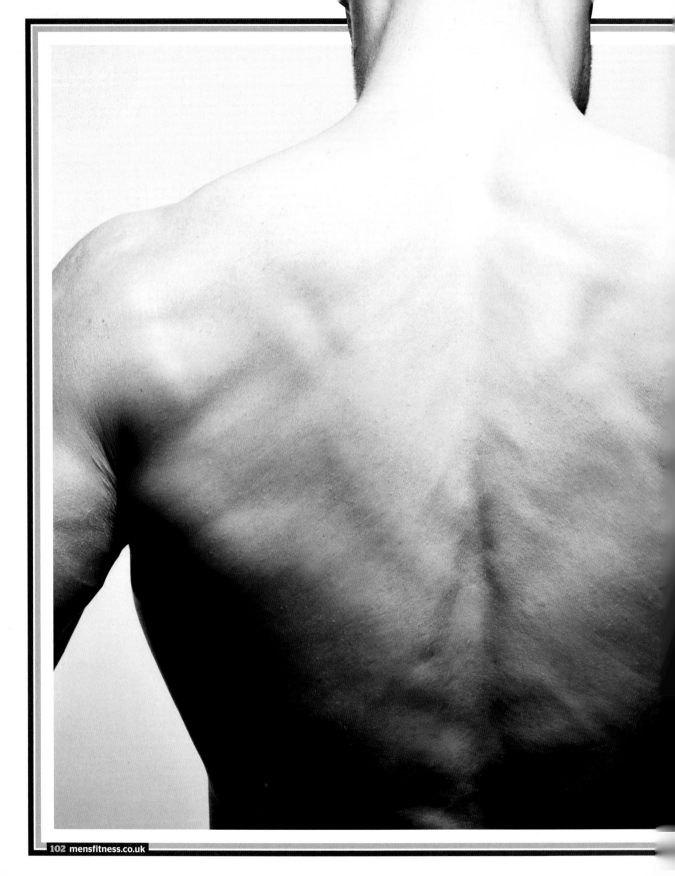

Back up plan

Get an impressively strong torso with these back workouts

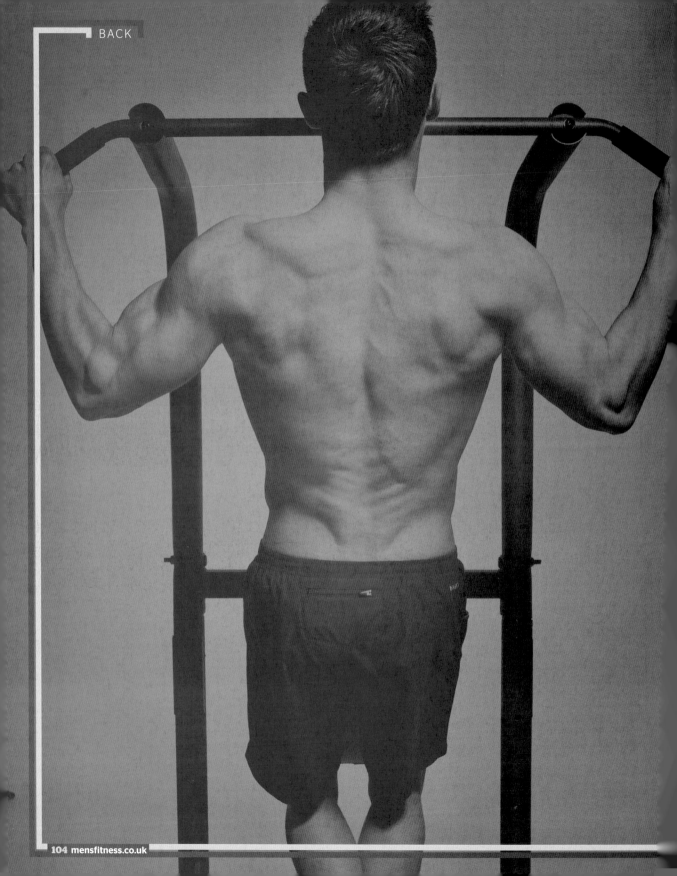

Back for good

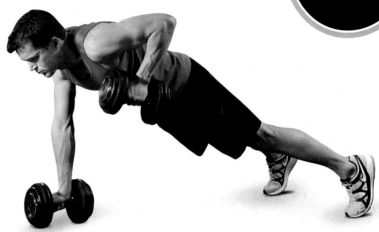

The back muscles don't get enough attention in most training programmes. Maybe it's because gym rats prefer to train the 'mirror muscles' in an attempt to look their best. Discover why this approach is all wrong and build a strong, impressive and injury-free body with these workouts.

How to do the workouts

Make gains fast with these four muscle-specific training plans

There are four workouts in this chapter. Each of these programmes is based on doing three sessions per week for a total of four weeks.

The first plan is a foundation workout designed for men of all athletic abilities, so make sure you start off by following this one rather than jumping straight into one of the three main workouts.

For those of you new to this type of exercise it will build a solid base from which you can launch into the more intense workouts. And even if you are a more experienced trainer, there's still much to gain from starting with the basics. It will help correct any muscular imbalances you may have, allow you to correct any poor form habits you may have picked up and let you master some simple movement patterns, including bodyweight moves, that you may have neglected during most of your previous training regimes.

ANATOMY OF THE MUSCLE GROUP BACK

Back

Your back contains a group of muscles that manipulate your shoulders and spine. Your trapezius muscles (traps) draw your shoulder blades up and together, and are aided by the rhomboids, which help to pull your shoulders back. Your latissimus dorsi (lats) lie down the sides of your back and are responsible for drawing your arms down from above, such as when you do a pull-up. Your erector spinae run down the middle of your lower back.

❶ **Trapezius**
❷ **Rhomboid**
❸ **Latissimus dorsi**
❹ **Erector spinae**

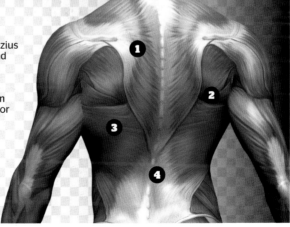

Foundation workout

It's easy to neglect your back muscles in favour of your chest and arms: after all, those are the muscles you can see every day in the mirror. But do so at your peril. A strong back will balance the muscles at the front of your body, creating all-over size and strength, so build a solid foundation with this workout that targets all the major muscles of the back.

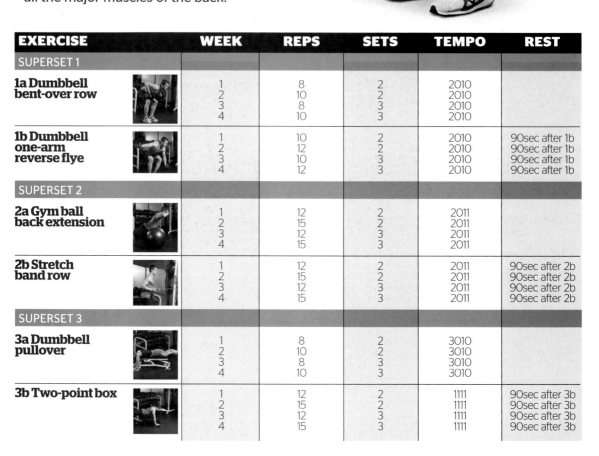

EXERCISE		WEEK	REPS	SETS	TEMPO	REST
SUPERSET 1						
1a Dumbbell bent-over row		1 2 3 4	8 10 8 10	2 2 3 3	2010 2010 2010 2010	
1b Dumbbell one-arm reverse flye		1 2 3 4	10 12 10 12	2 2 3 3	2010 2010 2010 2010	90sec after 1b 90sec after 1b 90sec after 1b 90sec after 1b
SUPERSET 2						
2a Gym ball back extension		1 2 3 4	12 15 12 15	2 2 3 3	2011 2011 2011 2011	
2b Stretch band row		1 2 3 4	12 15 12 15	2 2 3 3	2011 2011 2011 2011	90sec after 2b 90sec after 2b 90sec after 2b 90sec after 2b
SUPERSET 3						
3a Dumbbell pullover		1 2 3 4	8 10 8 10	2 2 3 3	3010 3010 3010 3010	
3b Two-point box		1 2 3 4	12 15 12 15	2 2 3 3	1111 1111 1111 1111	90sec after 3b 90sec after 3b 90sec after 3b 90sec after 3b

1a Reverse-grip dumbbell bent-over row

TARGETS
Biceps, back

WHY DO IT?
It's a great move to build
strength in your upper back and
biceps ahead of advancing to
heavier weights on a barbell.

HOW TO DO IT
● Stand tall holding a dumbbell
in each hand at arm's length with
palms facing away from you,
then bend forward from the hips,
keeping your core braced and
a natural arch in your back.
● Pull the weights in to your
chest, leading with your elbows.
● Slowly lower back to the start.

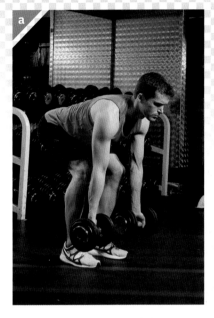
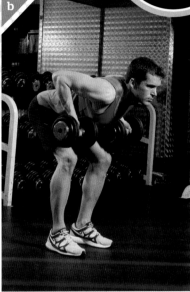

1b Dumbbell one-arm reverse flye

TARGETS
Rear deltoids, upper back

WHY DO IT?
Hit those often-neglected rear
delts and your upper back
with this unilateral move.

HOW TO DO IT
● Hold a dumbbell in each hand
and bend forward from the hips,
keeping your core braced.
● From there raise one arm up
and out to the side under control,
then return to the start and
repeat with your other arm.

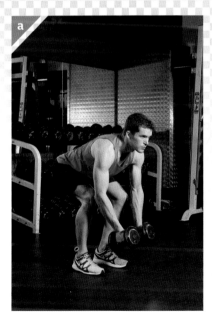
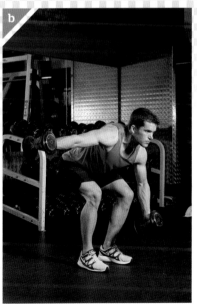

2a Gym ball back extension

TARGETS
Lower back

WHY DO IT?
You are only ever as strong as your weakest link and for most men it's their lower back, which this move will fix.

HOW TO DO IT
● Lie with your stomach on a gym ball with your hands by your temple.
● Raise your chest up and off the ball, pause at the top, squeeze your glutes, then return slowly to the start.

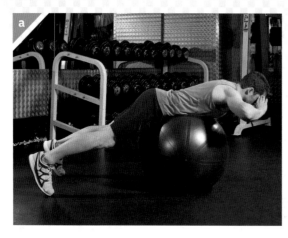
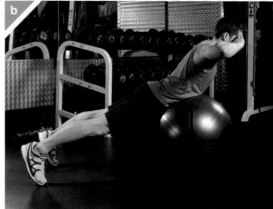

2b Stretch band rows

TARGETS
Upper back, biceps

WHY DO IT?
Hit all the major muscles of the back with this move.

HOW TO DO IT
● Stand tall with the handle of a stretch band in each hand after securing the middle of the band around a fixed object.
● Pull the handles towards your stomach, leading with your elbows and keeping your abs braced.
● Slowly return to the start.

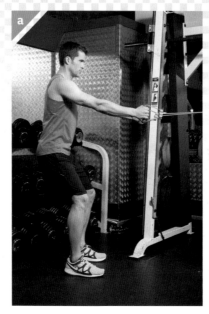
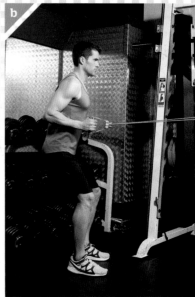

3a Dumbbell pullover

TARGETS

Chest, shoulders, upper back

WHY DO IT?

Although a single-joint move, this exercise works a large number of muscles, specifically the lats, lower chest and triceps.

HOW TO DO IT

● Lie flat on a bench with your head and shoulders supported and feet flat on the floor.
● Hold a dumbbell with both hands over your chest.
● Slowly lower the weight behind your head, keeping a slight bend in your elbows. Don't arch your back.
● Use your pecs to pull your arms back over your head to the start position.

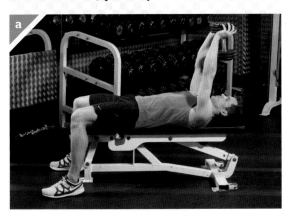
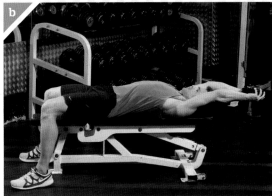

3b Two-point box

TARGETS

Back, core

WHY DO IT?

Work your back and core at the same time with this move that requires co-ordination and control.

HOW TO DO IT

● Start with your knees and hands on the floor with your core braced.
● Bring your left arm and right knee towards your stomach until they touch, then extend them forward until both are straight.
● Return to the start and repeat with the opposite arm and leg.

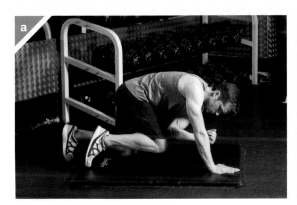
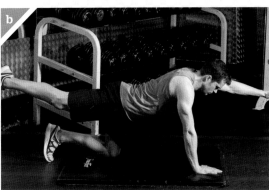

Workout one

↘ This tough workout works every muscle that runs down the back of your body, from traps to hamstrings – known as your posterior chain. A strong posterior chain will allow you to perform heavier lifts in every single major exercise and prevent injury and muscular imbalances.

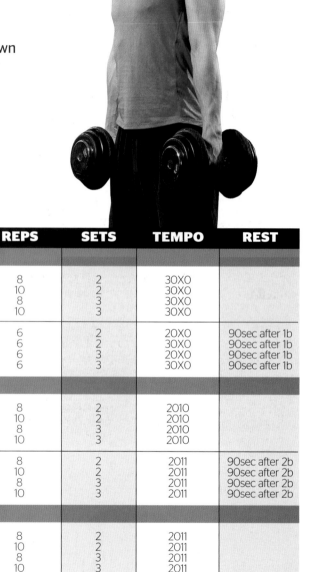

EXERCISE		WEEK	REPS	SETS	TEMPO	REST
SUPERSET 1						
1a Squat		1 2 3 4	8 10 8 10	2 2 3 3	30X0 30X0 30X0 30X0	
1b Pull-up		1 2 3 4	6 6 6 6	2 2 3 3	20X0 30X0 20X0 30X0	90sec after 1b 90sec after 1b 90sec after 1b 90sec after 1b
SUPERSET 2						
2a Good morning		1 2 3 4	8 10 8 10	2 2 3 3	2010 2010 2010 2010	
2b Seated reverse flye		1 2 3 4	8 10 8 10	2 2 3 3	2011 2011 2011 2011	90sec after 2b 90sec after 2b 90sec after 2b 90sec after 2b
SUPERSET 3						
3a Inverted row		1 2 3 4	8 10 8 10	2 2 3 3	2011 2011 2011 2011	
3b Shrug		1 2 3 4	10 12 10 12	2 2 3 3	2111 2111 2111 2111	90sec after 3b 90sec after 3b 90sec after 3b 90sec after 3b

1a Squat

TARGETS
Quads, glutes, hamstrings

WHY DO IT?
Although your legs are the obvious target, squats also work the lower back because it must stay strong to support correct form throughout the lift.

HOW TO DO IT
- Rest the bar against the back of your shoulders, holding it with an overhand grip slightly wider than your shoulders. Your feet should be shoulder-width apart.
- Lower yourself down, keeping your chest up, until your thighs are at least parallel to the floor. The deeper you can squat, the better.
- Drive back up through your heels without letting your knees roll inwards.

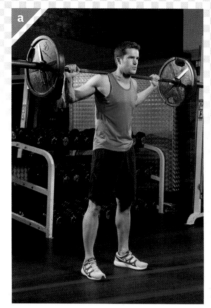
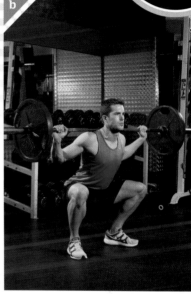

1b Pull-up

TARGETS
Upper back, core

WHY DO IT?
This is a seriously tough move because you control and lift your entire weight in conflict with gravity, but it'll build a strong, wide upper back, which helps create a wide, V-shaped torso.

HOW TO DO IT
- Grasp the bars with an overhand grip. If using a straight bar, your hands should be slightly wider than shoulder-width apart.
- Start from a dead hang with your arms fully extended.
- Pull yourself up by squeezing your lats together.
- Once your chin is higher than your hands, pause and then return to the start.

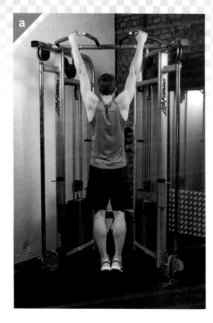
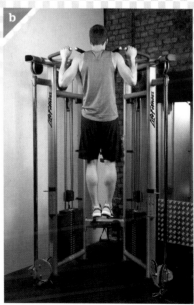

2a Good morning

WHY DO IT?

This move works the lower-back muscles as well as your hamstrings and glutes. Maintain perfect form throughout to prevent injury and start with a light bar.

HOW TO DO IT

● Stand tall holding a light barbell across the top of your shoulders.
● Brace your core, retract your shoulder blades and maintain a natural arch in your back.
● Feet should be between hip- and shoulder-width apart with a slight bend in your knees.
● Bend forward slowly from the hips, not the waist and lean forward as far as your hamstrings allow, but not past horizontal.
● Return to the start.

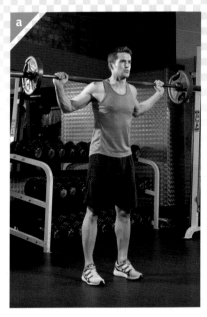
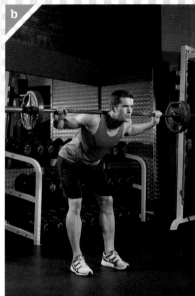

2b Seated reverse flye

TARGETS

Rear deltoids, upper back

WHY DO IT?

This move hits your rear delts, the back part of your shoulder muscles which is often ignored with standard shoulder moves, as well as your upper back.

HOW TO DO IT

● Lie on an incline bench with your chest against it, holding a dumbbell in each hand.
● Keeping a slight bend in your elbows, raise the weights out and to the sides.
● Slowly return to the start.

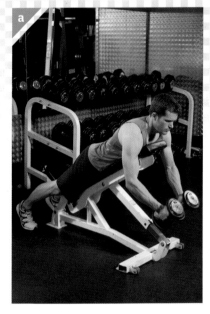
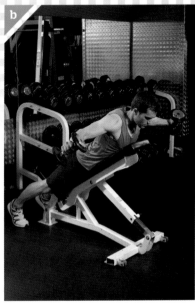

3a Inverted row

TARGETS
Back, biceps

WHY DO IT?
This move works all your major back muscles and your biceps. It will also build your grip strength without putting any pressure on your lower back.

HOW TO DO IT
● Set a Smith machine bar at about chest height. Lie underneath and hold it with an overhand grip.
● Keeping your hips in line with your torso, pull your body up to the bar until your touch it with your sternum.
● Lower yourself slowly back to the starting position.

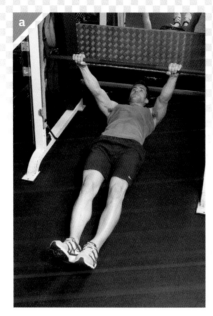
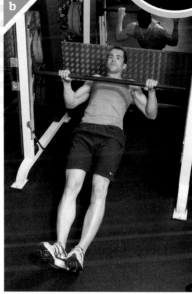

3b Shrug

TARGETS
Shoulders, traps

WHY DO IT?
Shrugs have a limited range of motion compared with most lifts. This means you can go really heavy on the weights to build big, strong traps and create wide shoulders.

HOW TO DO IT
● Stand between two heavy dumbbells, then squat down, grip the weights outside your hips and stand up, keeping your core braced.
● Shrug your shoulders up towards your ears, keeping your arms straight.
● Hold at the top before slowly lowering the weights again.

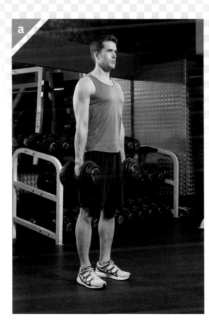
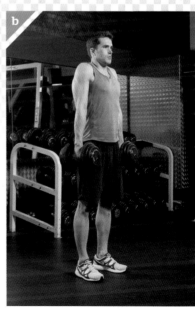

Workout two

⬊ The first superset – deadlifts and chin-ups – may seem to work the legs and biceps, but in fact both moves work the muscles of the back effectively. The other two supersets then work each part of the back individually so you can lift heavy to elicit the biggest growth hormone response possible.

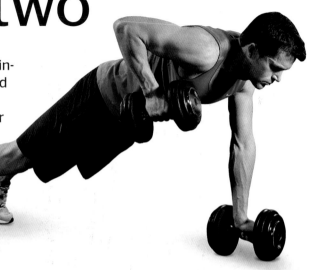

EXERCISE		WEEK	REPS	SETS	TEMPO	REST
SUPERSET 1						
1a Deadlift		1	8	2	20X0	
		2	6	3	20X0	
		3	8	3	20X0	
		4	10	3	20X0	
1b Chin-up		1	8	2	20X0	90sec after 1b
		2	8	3	30X0	90sec after 1b
		3	10	3	20X0	90sec after 1b
		4	10	3	30X0	90sec after 1b
SUPERSET 2						
2a Lat pull-down		1	10	2	2110	
		2	8	3	2110	
		3	10	3	2110	
		4	12	3	2110	
2b Bent-over flye		1	10	2	2110	90sec after 2b
		2	8	3	2110	90sec after 2b
		3	10	3	2110	90sec after 2b
		4	12	3	2110	90sec after 2b
SUPERSET 3						
3a Renegade row		1	10	2	1010	
		2	8	3	1010	
		3	10	3	1010	
		4	12	3	1010	
3b Gym ball back extension		1	15	2	2111	90sec after 3b
		2	12	3	2111	90sec after 3b
		3	12	3	2111	75sec after 3b
		4	15	3	2111	75sec after 3b

1a Deadlift

TARGETS
Total body

WHY DO IT?
Performed correctly, this is one of the best exercises for developing a strong and supportive lower back, making you stronger in almost every other full-body lift.

HOW TO DO IT
- Grip the bar just outside your knees with your core braced and your back flat.
- Use your glutes to power the initial lift, pushing down through your heels.
- As the bar passes your knees, push your hips forward. Return to the start.
- Keep your shoulders back throughout the move.

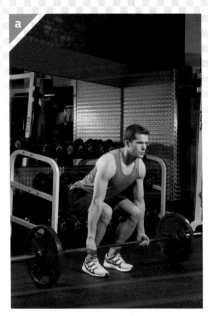
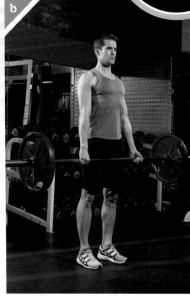

1b Chin-up

TARGETS
Biceps, upper back

WHY DO IT?
This tough bodyweight move will get your heart rate up and release growth hormones into your blood.

HOW TO DO IT
- Grab the bars with an underhand grip. If using a straight bar your hands should be slightly wider than shoulder-width apart.
- Start from a dead hang with your arms fully extended.
- Pull yourself up by squeezing your lats together.
- Once your chin is higher than your hands pause briefly, before slowly lowering yourself back to the start.

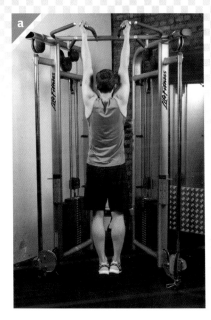
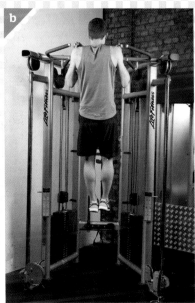

2a Lat pull-down

TARGETS
Upper back, core

WHY DO IT?
This works the same muscles as the pull-up but the machine allows you to adjust the resistance easily.

HOW TO DO IT
● Sit on the seat and take an overhand, wide-grip on the bar.
● Look forward, retract your shoulder blades and keep your torso upright.
● Pull the bar down in front of you until it reaches your upper chest. Don't lean back to aid the movement.
● Squeeze your lats at the bottom of the move and return the bar slowly to the top.

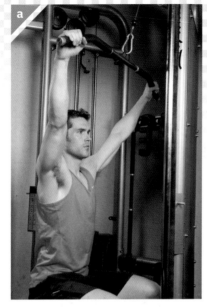
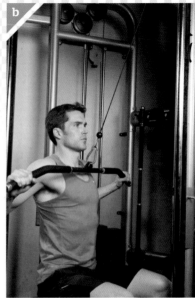

2b Bent-over flye

TARGETS
Rear deltoids, upper back

WHY DO IT?
Hit those often-neglected rear delts and your upper back with this unilateral move.

HOW TO DO IT
● Hold a dumbbell in each hand and bend forward from the hips.
● Keeping a slight bend in your elbows, raise your arms up and out to the sides, then return to the start.

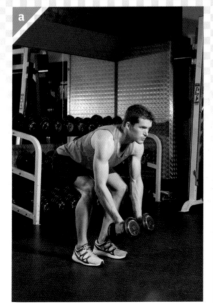
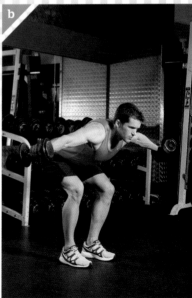

3a Renegade row

TARGETS
Back, biceps, core

WHY DO IT?
Pulling the weights from the floor discourages poor form because

you can't use momentum.

HOW TO DO IT
● Place a pair of dumbbells on the floor shoulder-width apart and assume a press-up position over them with

your body in a straight line.
● Shift your weight to the left side of your body, and pull the right dumbbell towards your hip in a rowing fashion. Return it to the floor slowly.
● Repeat on the other side.

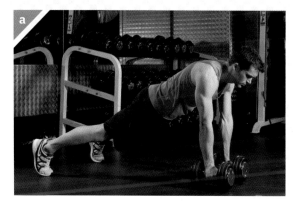
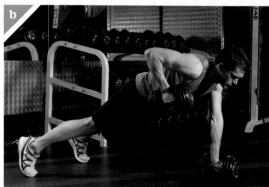

3b Gym ball back extension

TARGETS
Lower back

WHY DO IT?
It will strengthen your lower

back, which will help your perform heavier lifts better.

HOW TO DO IT
● Lie on your stomach

on a gym ball with your hands by your temples.
● Raise your chest up and off the ball, pause at the top, then return slowly to the start.

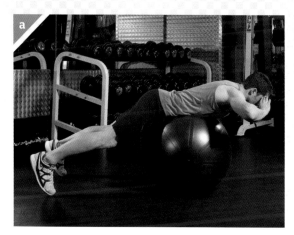
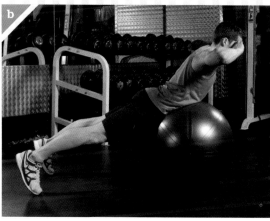

Workout three

↘ This session focuses at first on the powerhouse muscles of the upper back – traps, rhomboids and lats – with some hard-hitting compound and isolation moves. Then it moves on to the often-neglected lower-back muscles with some tough bodyweight moves that require balance and co-ordination.

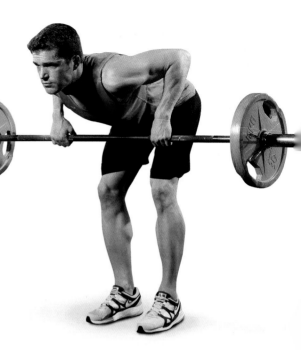

EXERCISE	WEEK	REPS	SETS	TEMPO	REST
SUPERSET 1					
1a Bent-over row	1	8	2	20X0	
	2	8	3	20X0	
	3	10	3	20X0	
	4	10	4	20X0	
1b Upright row	1	10	2	20X0	90sec after 1b
	2	10	3	20X0	90sec after 1b
	3	12	3	20X0	90sec after 1b
	4	12	4	20X0	90sec after 1b
SUPERSET 2					
2a One-arm pull-down	1	12	2	2110	
	2	10	3	2110	
	3	12	3	2110	
	4	12	4	2110	
2b Standing cable row	1	12	2	2110	90sec after 2b
	2	10	3	2110	90sec after 2b
	3	12	3	2110	75sec after 2b
	4	12	4	2110	75sec after 2b
SUPERSET 3					
3a Two-point box	1	15	2	2020	
	2	12	3	2020	
	3	15	3	2020	
	4	12	4	2020	
3b Aquaman	1	15	2	2020	75sec after 3b
	2	12	3	2020	75sec after 3b
	3	15	3	2020	60sec after 3b
	4	12	4	2020	60sec after 3b

1a Bent-over row

TARGETS
Upper back, biceps, core

WHY DO IT?
This move works the powerhouse muscles of the upper back – traps, lats, rhomboids and rear deltoids – as well as your core, which help keep your torso stable.

HOW TO DO IT
● Start with your core braced, back straight, shoulder blades retracted and knees slightly bent.
● Lean forward from the hips and grip the bar with your hands just wider than shoulder-width apart letting them hang at knee level.
● Pull the bar up almost to your chest, retracting your shoulder blades, then lower it slowly back to the start.

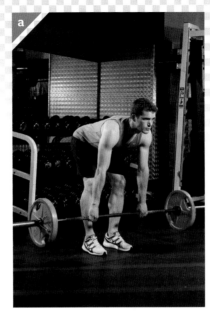
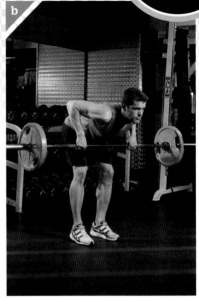

1b Upright row

TARGETS
Shoulders, traps

WHY DO IT?
This move mainly works your traps and shoulders to help craft a strong and wide torso.

HOW TO DO IT
● Stand tall holding a barbell with an overhand grip slightly narrower than shoulder-width.
● Shrug the bar up towards your chin, leading with your elbows.
● Slowly lower the bar back to the start.

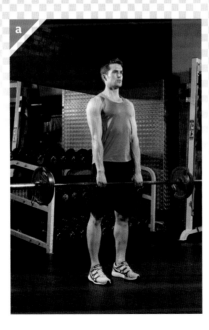
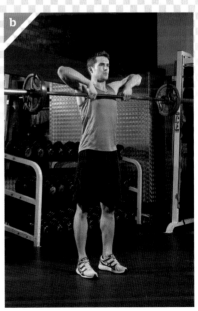

2a One-arm pull-down

TARGETS
Upper back, biceps

WHY DO IT?
Working each arm independently
will ensure balanced gains.

HOW TO DO IT
● Sit on the seat and hold a
D-handle with one hand.
● Look forward, retract
your shoulder blades and
keep your torso upright.
● Pull the handle down in front
of you until it reaches your upper
chest. Don't attempt to aid the
movement by leaning back.
● Squeeze your lats at the
bottom of the move and return
the bar slowly to the top.

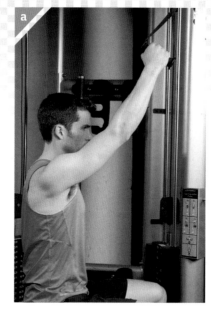
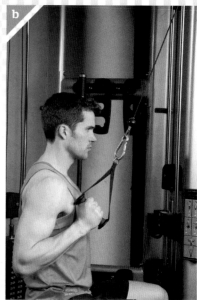

2b Standing cable row

TARGETS
Biceps, upper back

WHY DO IT?
Hitting your back muscles while
standing also works your core, so
you get big muscle-mass benefits.

HOW TO DO IT
● Stand tall with a slight
bend in your knees, holding a
double-D handle attached to
the middle pulley of a cable
machine with a neutral grip.
● Ensure that there is tension
in the cable before you begin.
● Pull the handle in to your chest,
keeping upper-body movement
to a minimum, and squeeze
your shoulder blades together.
● Return slowly to the start.

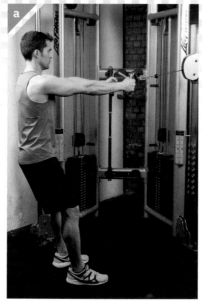
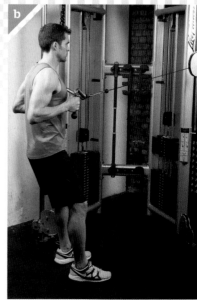

3a Two-point box

TARGETS
Back, core

WHY DO IT?
This works your deep-lying core and lower-back muscles that are often neglected and will improve balance and co-ordination.

HOW TO DO IT
● Start with your knees and hands on the floor with your core braced.
● Bring your left arm and right knee towards your stomach until they touch, then extend them forward until both are straight.
● Return to the start and repeat with the opposite arm and leg.

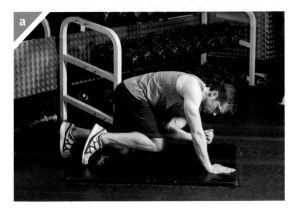
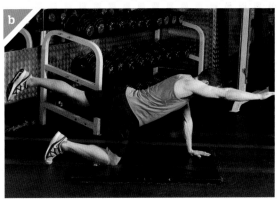

3b Aquaman

TARGET
Lower back

WHY DO IT?
It's great move for the stabilising muscles around your spine.

HOW TO DO IT
● Lie flat on your front with legs and arms fully extended.
● Raise your left arm and right leg up, holding briefly at the top before lowering.
● Raise your right arm and left leg and keep alternating with each rep.

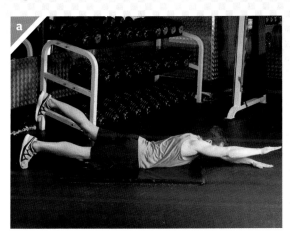
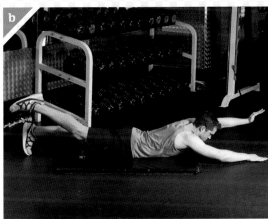

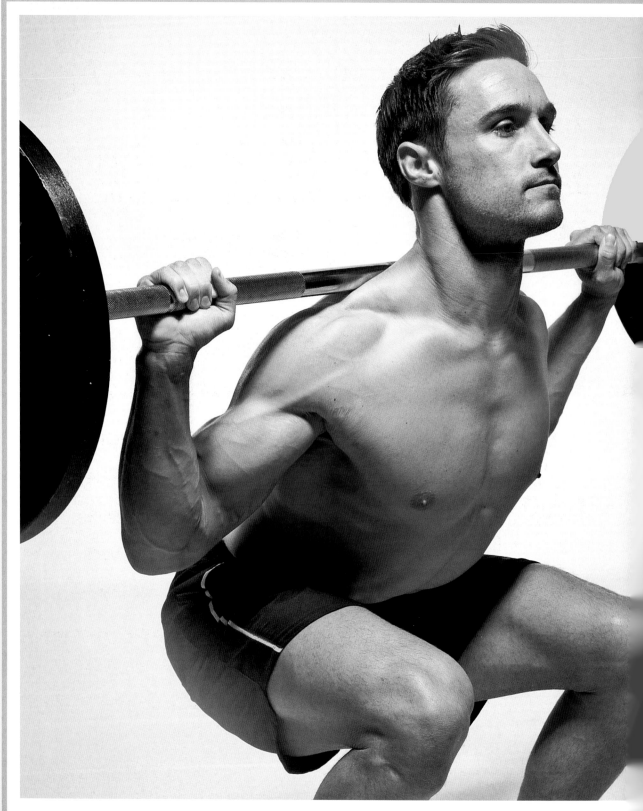

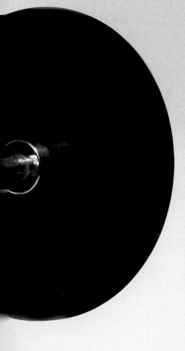

Build big legs

Get strong and impressive quads, hams and calves

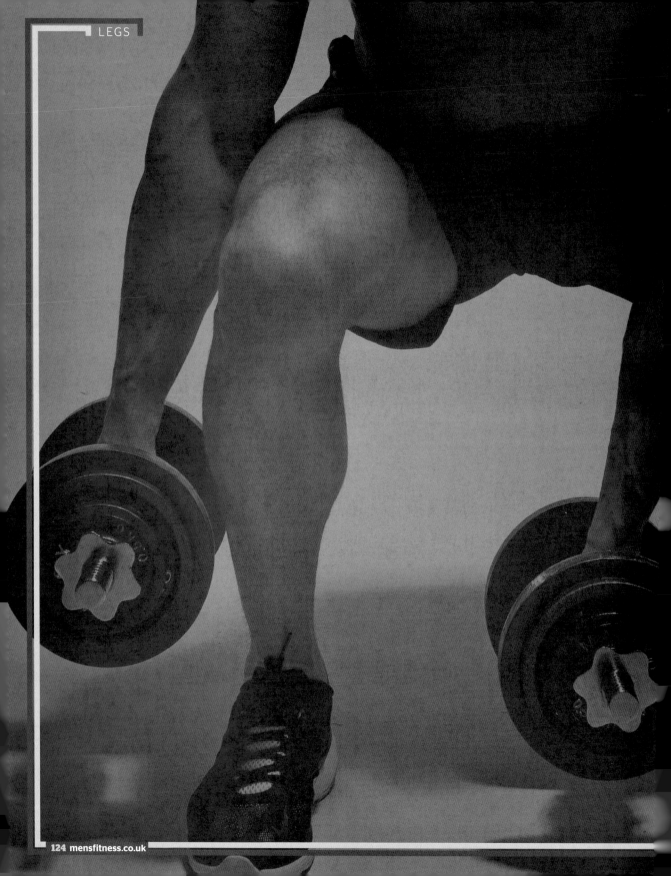

Getting a leg up

When trying to build a cover model body it's tempting to overlook your legs in favour of working those muscles you see every day in the mirror, such as your shoulders, chest, arms and abs. But neglecting your powerhouse lower-body muscles is the biggest mistake you can make. Training your legs hard with heavy weights releases a number of growth hormones into your system, which promote muscle growth and burn fat.

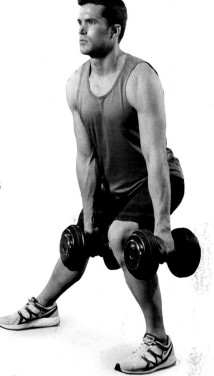

How to do the workouts

Make gains fast with these four muscle-specific training plans

There are four workouts in this chapter. Each of these programmes is based on doing three sessions per week for a total of four weeks.

The first plan is a foundation workout designed for men of all athletic abilities, so make sure you start off by following this one rather than jumping straight into one of the three main workouts.

For those of you new to this type of exercise it will build a solid base from which you can launch into the more intense workouts. And even if you are a more experienced trainer, there's still much to gain from starting with the basics. It will help correct any muscular imbalances you may have, allow you to correct any poor form habits you may have picked up and let you master some simple movement patterns, including bodyweight moves, that you may have neglected during most of your previous training regimes.

ANATOMY OF THE MUSCLE GROUP LEGS

Legs

Your glutes extend your hip joint, while the quads and hamstrings move the knee to straighten and bend your leg respectively. The two lower-leg muscles, which make up your calf, act on your ankle to move your foot.

❶ **Quadriceps** *(on front of leg)*
(comprising rectus femoris, vastus medialis, vastus intermedius and vastus lateralis)
❷ **Gluteus maximus**
❸ **Hamstring**
(comprising biceps femoris, semitendinosus and semimembranosus)
❹ **Gastrocnemius**
❺ **Soleus**

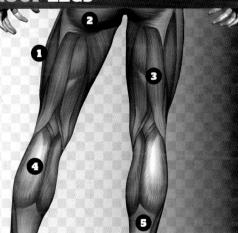

Foundation workout

Training your legs will pack on muscles not just in your lower body but everywhere else too. The trouble is that most of the best leg exercise are fairly complex so it's well worth learning the movement patterns for these key moves first. Dumbbells are a great way to get to grips with the big lifts, and this workout uses them to get your muscles used to what lies ahead, then ends with some explosive exercises to shock your muscles into growth.

EXERCISE	WEEK	REPS	SETS	TEMPO	REST
SUPERSET 1					
1a Dumbbell squat	1 2 3 4	8 10 8 10	2 2 3 3	20X0 20X0 20X0 20X0	
1b Dumbbell lateral lunge	1 2 3 4	10 12 10 12	2 2 3 3	2010 2010 2010 2010	90sec after 1b 90sec after 1b 90sec after 1b 90sec after 1b
SUPERSET 2					
2a Dumbbell step-up	1 2 3 4	10 12 10 12	2 2 3 3	1010 1010 1010 1010	
2b Box jump	1 2 3 4	10 12 10 12	2 2 3 3	X X X X	90sec after 2b 90sec after 2b 90sec after 2b 90sec after 2b
SUPERSET 3					
3a Glute bridge	1 2 3 4	12 15 12 15	2 2 3 3	1111 1111 1111 1111	
3b Mountain climber	1 2 3 4	10 12 10 12	2 2 3 3	X X X X	90sec after 3b 90sec after 3b 90sec after 3b 90sec after 3b

1a Dumbbell squat

TARGETS
Quads, hams, glutes

WHY DO IT?
If you struggle to maintain good form with a barbell, performing squats with a dumbbell can help you learn to do the move safely.

HOW TO DO IT
- Stand tall with feet shoulder-width apart, holding a dumbbell in each hand at your side.
- With you core braced and a natural arch in your back, squat down until your thighs are at least parallel to the floor, keeping your knees in line with your toes.
- Push back up through your heels to complete the move.

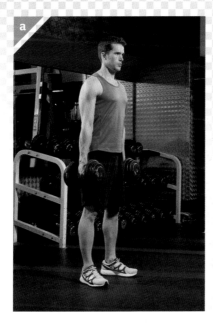
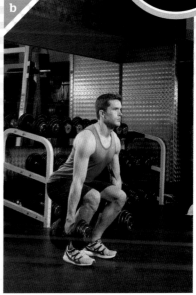

1b Dumbbell lateral lunge

TARGETS
Hams, glutes, adductors

WHY DO IT?
This move targets the often-forgotten inner thigh muscles. Ignoring them can lead to muscular imbalances and injury, while strengthening them will improve all lower-body lifts.

HOW TO DO IT
- Stand tall with feet close together, holding a dumbbell in each hand.
- Keeping your core braced, take a big step to one side and lower your body down towards the leading leg, with your knee in line with your toes.
- Push back off the leading leg and repeat the other side.

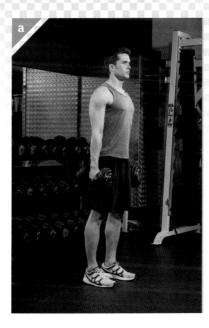
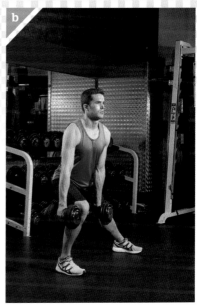

2a Dumbbell step-up

TARGETS
Quads, hams, glutes, calves

WHY DO IT?
Your legs are used to walking up steps daily, but adding extra weight shocks them into growing bigger and stronger.

HOW TO DO IT
● Stand in front of a bench set below knee height with a dumbbell in each hand.
● Step up on to the bench, then reverse the movement back down.
● For the next rep, step up with the other leg.

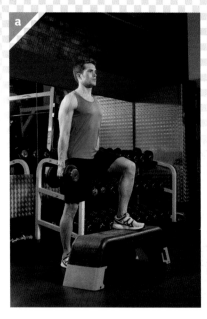
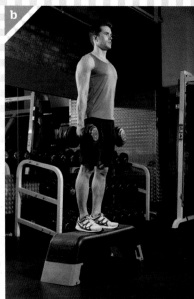

2b Box jump

TARGETS
Quads, hams, glutes core

WHY DO IT?
This plyometric move is great for raising your heart rate and building explosive speed and power.

HOW TO DO IT
● Stand in front of a bench set below knee height.
● Bend down, then jump explosively up on to the bench.
● Step back down and repeat.

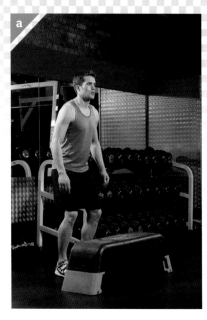
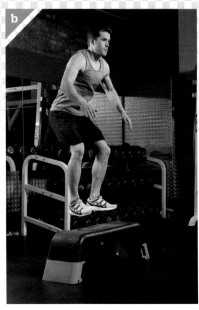

3a Glute bridge

TARGETS
Glutes

WHY DO IT?
To make all lower-body lifts easier.

HOW TO DO IT
● Lie flat on your back with your arms by your sides.
● Place both feet on the floor, directly underneath your knees,
then raise your lower back and glutes off the floor, keeping your core braced throughout.
● Hold at the top position briefly, then lower back to the start.

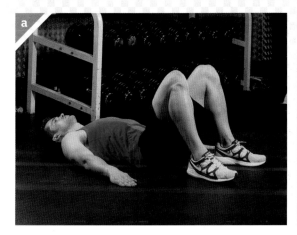
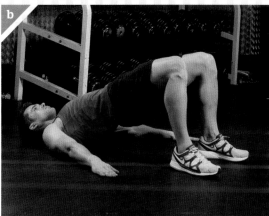

3b Mountain climber

TARGETS
Core, legs

WHY DO IT?
It's a great move for getting your
heart rate high and working the fast-twitch muscles of your legs.

HOW TO DO IT
● Start in a press-up position.
● With your core braced, bring your right knee up to your chest.
● Straighten your leg again, then repeat with the other leg. That's one rep.

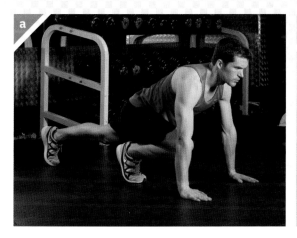
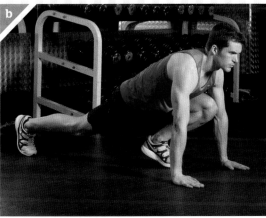

Workout one

The first two supersets in this session alternate between hitting your quads and your hamstrings, the two major muscles of the leg. Working these antagonistic muscle groups in turn allows you to lift heavy and then recover before hitting them again. The final superset targets your calves to help build solid lower legs.

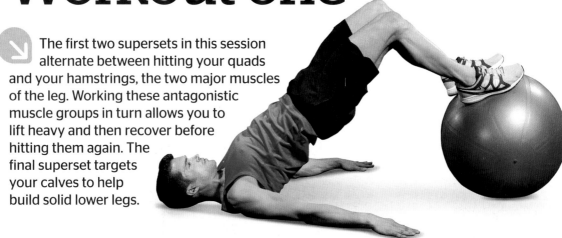

EXERCISE		WEEK	REPS	SETS	TEMPO	REST
SUPERSET 1						
1a Squat		1	8	2	20X0	
		2	10	2	20X0	
		3	8	3	30X0	
		4	10	3	30X0	
1b Gym ball leg curl		1	10	2	20X0	90sec after 1b
		2	12	2	20X0	90sec after 1b
		3	10	3	30X0	90sec after 1b
		4	12	3	30X0	90sec after 1b
SUPERSET 2						
2a Hack squat		1	8	2	20X0	
		2	10	2	20X0	
		3	8	3	30X0	
		4	10	3	30X0	
2b Romanian deadlift		1	8	2	2010	90sec after 2b
		2	10	2	2010	90sec after 2b
		3	8	3	3010	90sec after 2b
		4	10	3	3010	90sec after 2b
SUPERSET 3						
3a Standing calf raise		1	10	2	2111	
		2	12	2	2111	
		3	10	3	2111	
		4	12	3	2111	
3b Dumbbell side step-up		1	10	2	1010	90sec after 3b
		2	12	2	1010	90sec after 3b
		3	12	3	1010	90sec after 3b
		4	15	3	1010	90sec after 3b

1a Squat

TARGETS
Quads, glutes, hamstrings

WHY DO IT?
This targets all the major leg muscles as well as releasing growth-boosting hormones.

HOW TO DO IT
● Hold the bar against the back of your shoulders, using an overhand grip slightly wider than your shoulders. Your feet should be wider than shoulder-width apart.
● Slowly squat down, keeping your chest up, until your thighs are at least parallel to the floor. The deeper you can squat, the better.
● Drive back up through your heels, keeping your knees in line with your feet. At the top push forward with your hips and squeeze your glutes, then repeat.

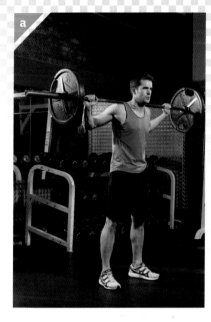
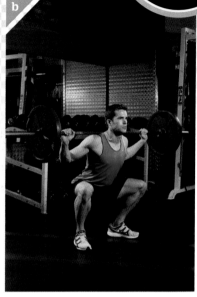

1b Gym ball leg curl

TARGETS
Hamstring, glutes

WHY DO IT?
You may only be using your own bodyweight, but this tough move hits your hamstrings hard.

HOW TO DO IT
● Lie with your head, shoulders and upper back on a gym mat and your feet together on top of a gym ball. Your body should form a straight line from head to heels.

● Keeping your back straight, raise your hips and drag the ball towards your backside with your heels.
● Pause briefly at the top of the move, then slowly return to the start.

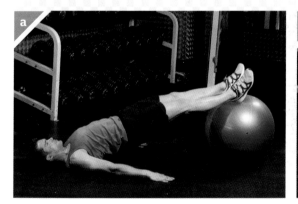
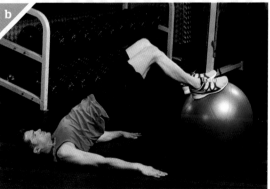

2a Hack squat

TARGETS
Quads, hams, glutes

WHY DO IT?
Holding the bar behind your body places less strain on your back and greater emphasis on your powerful quad muscles.

HOW TO DO IT
● Stand in front of a barbell with your feet shoulder-width apart. Squat down and grasp the bar with an overhand grip. .
● Keeping your feet flat on the floor, knees in line with your toes, head up, core braced and a neutral arch in your back, push through you heels until you're fully upright.
● Lower until your thighs are at least parallel to the floor, then stand back up.

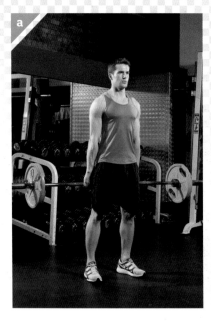
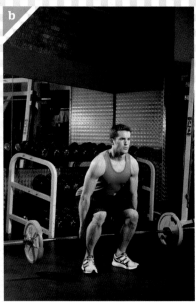

2b Romanian deadlift

WHY DO IT?
This is one of the best moves for building muscle mass on the backs of your legs. Perfect form is vital to prevent injury.

HOW TO DO IT
● Stand tall with feet shoulder-width apart holding a barbell with an overhand grip just outside your hips. Keep your shoulder blades retracted, your torso upright, your core braced and a natural arch in your back.
● Initiate the move by slowly leaning forward from the hips, not the waist, and lower the bar slowly down the front of your shins until you feel a good stretch in your hamstrings.
● Reverse the move back to the start and push your hips forward to reset the start position.

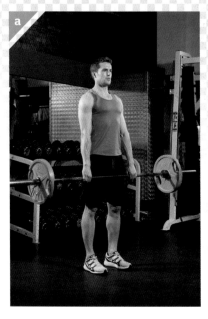
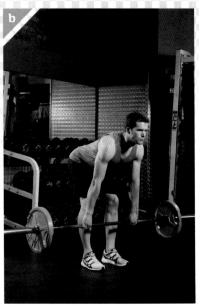

3a Standing calf raise

TARGETS
Calves

WHY DO IT?
The calves are used to working hard every day so shock them into growing with heavy weights

HOW TO DO IT
● Stand on the edge of a platform with a dumbbell in one hand, while the other holds on to a fixed object for support.
● Go up onto your tiptoes, keeping your body stable.
● Pause briefly, then return to the start, ensuring your heels go below the platform so you go through a full range of motion.

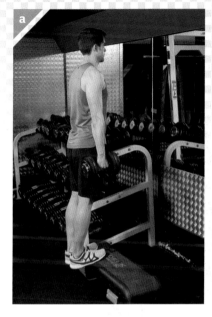
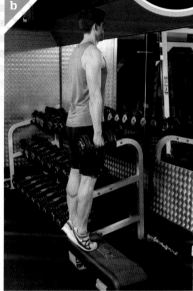

3b Dumbbell side step-up

TARGETS
Quads, glutes, adductors, calves

WHY DO IT?
You'll work the insides of your thighs as well as your powerhouse lower-body muscles.

HOW TO DO IT
● Stand tall side-on to a bench set at lower than knee height holding a dumbbell in each hand.
● Step up sideways on to the bench.
● Reverse the move back down, then repeat.

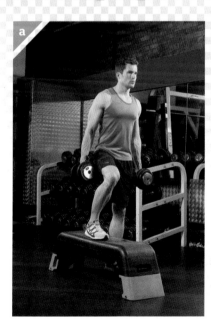
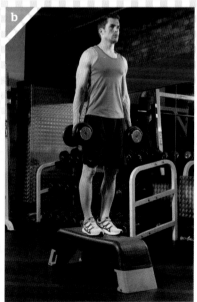

Workout two

↘ These tough supersets will blitz your glutes, hams, quads and calves from every possible angle, which is the best way to shock your muscles into growing back bigger and stronger. These moves also work your core really effectively, so you'll carve a rock-solid six-pack as a bonus.

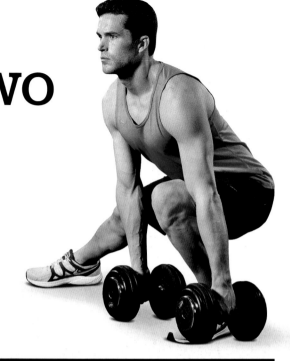

EXERCISE		WEEK	REPS	SETS	TEMPO	REST
SUPERSET 1						
1a Deadlift		1	8	2	20X0	
		2	6	3	20X0	
		3	8	3	20X0	
		4	10	3	20X0	
1b Barbell lunges		1	10	2	2010	90sec after 1b
		2	8	3	2010	90sec after 1b
		3	10	3	2010	90sec after 1b
		4	12	3	2010	90sec after 1b
SUPERSET 2						
2a Back of steel		1	6	2	2121	
		2	4	3	2121	
		3	6	3	2121	
		4	8	3	2121	
2b Dumbbell lunge and touch		1	12	2	1111	90sec after 2b
		2	10	3	1111	90sec after 2b
		3	12	3	1111	90sec after 2b
		4	14	3	1111	90sec after 2b
SUPERSET 3						
3a Jump lunge		1	12	2	X	
		2	10	3	X	
		3	12	3	X	
		4	14	3	X	
3b Gym ball supine calf raise		1	15	2	2111	90sec after 3b
		2	12	3	2111	90sec after 3b
		3	15	3	2111	90sec after 3b
		4	20	3	2111	90sec after 3b

1a Deadlift

TARGETS
Total body

WHY DO IT?
Along with squats, deadlifts are among the most important moves for adding size and strength to your lower body.

HOW TO DO IT
● Grip the bar just outside your knees with your core braced, your shoulders retracted and over the bar and your back flat.
● Use your glutes to power the initial lift, pushing down through your heels.
● Keep the bar close to your body and, as it passes your knees, push your hips forward. Keep your shoulders back throughout the move.

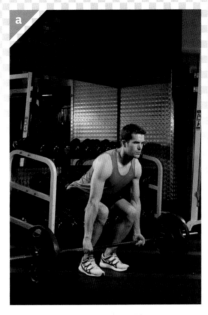
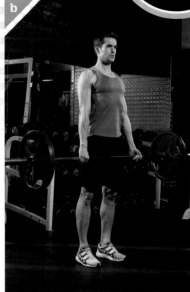

1b Barbell lunge

TARGETS
Hams, glutes, quads, core

WHY DO IT?
Lunges work the powerful lower-body muscles and also involve the adductors, hip flexors and many other stabilising muscles, including your core.

HOW TO DO IT
● Stand tall with a barbell resting on the back of your shoulders. Point your elbows behind you to retract your shoulder blades and keep your back upright and core braced throughout.
● Take a big step forward, making sure your knee does not go beyond your front foot. Lower until both knees are bent at 90°, then push off your front foot to return to the start position.

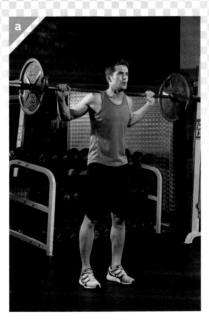
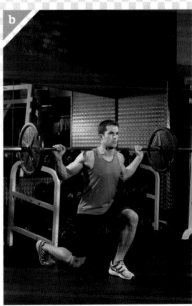

2a Back of steel

TARGETS
Legs, core, shoulders

WHY DO IT?
Not only does this move work your shoulders, it also really taxes your abs and legs to hold the squat position whilst lifting. Start with light dumbbells.

HOW TO DO IT
● Stand tall with a dumbbell in each hand with both arms directly above your head.
● Squat down, keeping your arms straight up, until your thighs are parallel to the ground.
● Once there, lower the weights down to shoulder height then press them back up.

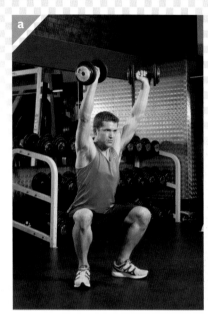
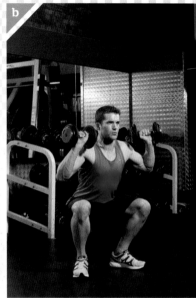

2b Dumbbell lateral lunge and touch

TARGETS
Hamstrings, inner thighs

WHY DO IT?
This move targets the often-forgotten inner thigh muscles.

HOW TO DO IT
● Stand tall with feet close together, holding a dumbbell in each hand.
● Keeping your core braced and head looking forward, take a big step to one side and lower your body down towards the leading leg, with your knee in line with your toes.
● Reach down with the dumbbells as far as you can comfortably go, keeping your back straight. It's fine if they touch the floor.
● Push back off the leading leg and repeat the other side.

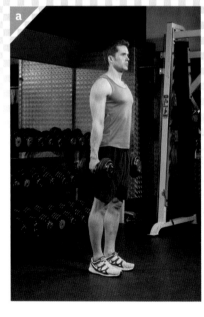
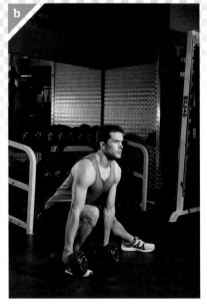

3a Jump lunge

TARGETS
Hams, glutes, quads, core

WHY DO IT?
These require explosive power to jump high enough to switch legs and land straight back into a lunge, leading to rapid muscle growth.

HOW TO DO IT
● Start in a lunge, then jump straight up.
● Switch legs in mid-air to land with your other foot forward.
● Descend straight into a lunge and repeat.

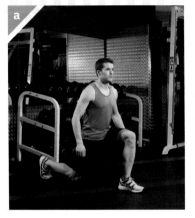
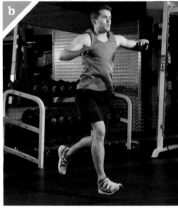
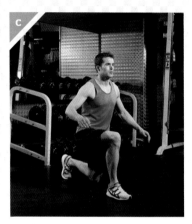

3b Gym ball supine calf raise

TARGETS
Calves

WHY DO IT?
This is a great move for isolating the hard-to-grow calves.

HOW TO DO IT
● Lie with your back supported on a gym ball with feet flat on the floor.
● Rise up onto your tiptoes, pause at the top, then return to the start.

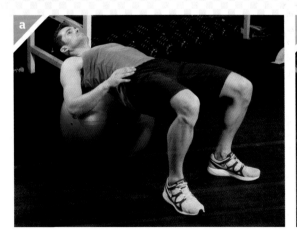
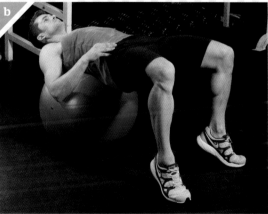

Workout three

The final workout begins with some twists on the two classic leg lifts, and it's these slight tweaks that keep your muscles guessing so they have no choice but to keep getting bigger and stronger. You'll then work the legs and shoulders before hitting the hard-to-grow calves with tough back-to-back moves.

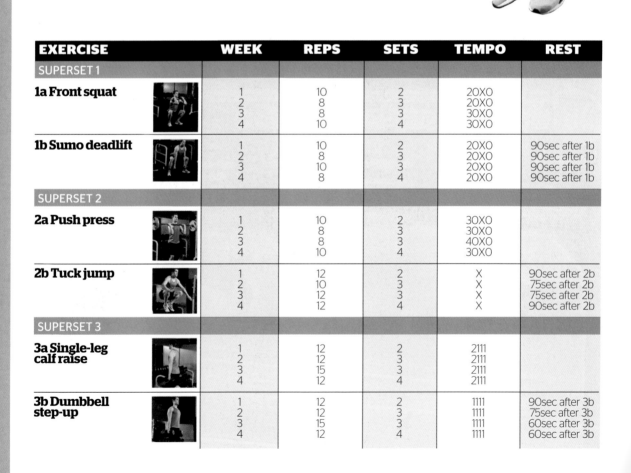

EXERCISE		WEEK	REPS	SETS	TEMPO	REST
SUPERSET 1						
1a Front squat		1 2 3 4	10 8 8 10	2 3 3 4	20X0 20X0 30X0 30X0	
1b Sumo deadlift		1 2 3 4	10 8 10 8	2 3 3 4	20X0 20X0 20X0 20X0	90sec after 1b 90sec after 1b 90sec after 1b 90sec after 1b
SUPERSET 2						
2a Push press		1 2 3 4	10 8 8 10	2 3 3 4	30X0 30X0 40X0 30X0	
2b Tuck jump		1 2 3 4	12 10 12 12	2 3 3 4	X X X X	90sec after 2b 75sec after 2b 75sec after 2b 90sec after 2b
SUPERSET 3						
3a Single-leg calf raise		1 2 3 4	12 12 15 12	2 3 3 4	2111 2111 2111 2111	
3b Dumbbell step-up		1 2 3 4	12 12 15 12	2 3 3 4	1111 1111 1111 1111	90sec after 3b 75sec after 3b 60sec after 3b 60sec after 3b

1a Front squat

TARGETS
Quads, glutes, hams, core

WHY DO IT?
Resting the bar on the front of your shoulders is an excellent way to target your quads while protecting the lower back.

HOW TO DO IT
- Stand with your feet shoulder-width apart and rest the bar on the front of your shoulders, gripping it with your elbows pointing forward.
- Maintain a natural arch in your back and core braced throughout the move.
- Squat down until your thighs are at least parallel to the floor.
- Push back up through your heels to the start position.

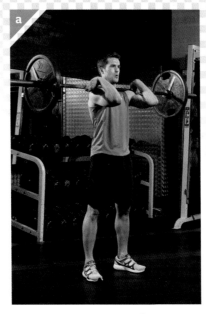
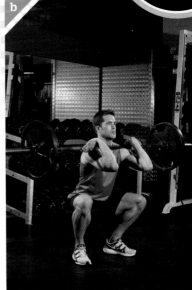

1b Sumo deadlift

TARGETS
Total body

WHY DO IT?
The wider stance of the sumo deadlift recruits the glutes, one of the strongest muscles in your body, more than the classic deadlift does.

HOW TO DO IT
- Stand behind the bar with your feet wider than shoulder-width apart and your toes pointing outwards.
- Squat down and grip the bar with your hands shoulder-width apart.
- Keeping a natural arch in your lower back, drive with your legs and push your hips forward, lifting the bar to your thighs.
- Reverse the motion, returning the bar to the floor.

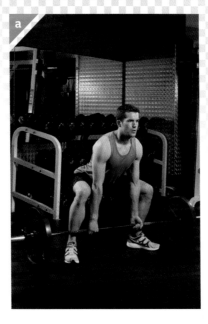
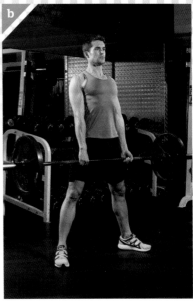

2a Push press

TARGETS
Legs, core, shoulders

WHY DO IT?
Using your legs to assist the move allows you to lift heavier, priming your muscles for growth.

HOW TO DO IT
● Stand with feet shoulder-width apart with the bar resting across the front of your shoulders.
● Bend your knees slightly then stand up straight to generate momentum. As you do, press the bar directly overhead.
● Slowly lower the weight back to the start position.

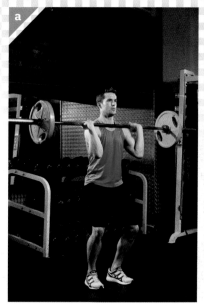
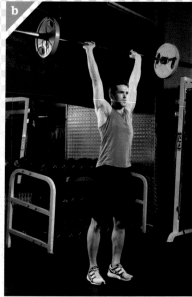

2b Tuck jump

TARGETS
Total body

WHY DO IT?
Fire up your heart rate and get your muscles warm with this plyometric bodyweight move.

HOW TO DO IT
● Stand tall with feet closer than hip width apart.
● Bend your knees, then jump up, tucking your knees up in front of you.
● Land and repeat.

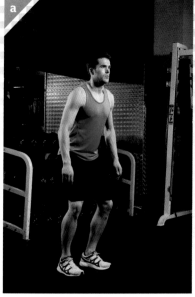
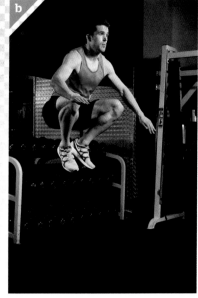

Single-leg calf raise

TARGETS
Calves

WHY DO IT?
Working your calves individually makes them work harder and ensures balanced gains

HOW TO DO IT
● Stand with one foot on the edge of a platform with a dumbbell in one hand, while the other holds on to a fixed object for support.
● Go up on to your tiptoes, keeping your body stable.
● Pause briefly, then return to the start, ensuring your heel goes below the platform so you go through a full range of motion.

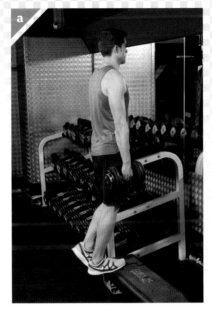
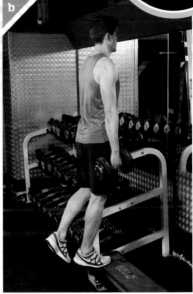

Dumbbell step-up

TARGETS
Quads, hams, glutes

WHY DO IT?
Your legs are used to walking up steps daily, but adding extra weight shocks them into growing bigger and stronger.

HOW TO DO IT
● Stand in front of a bench set below knee height with a dumbbell in each hand.
● Step up on to the bench, then reverse the movement back to the start.
● For the next rep, step up with the other leg.

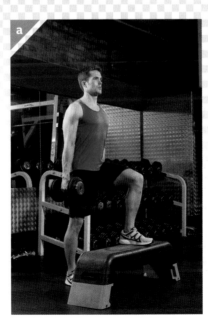
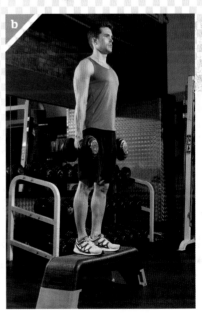

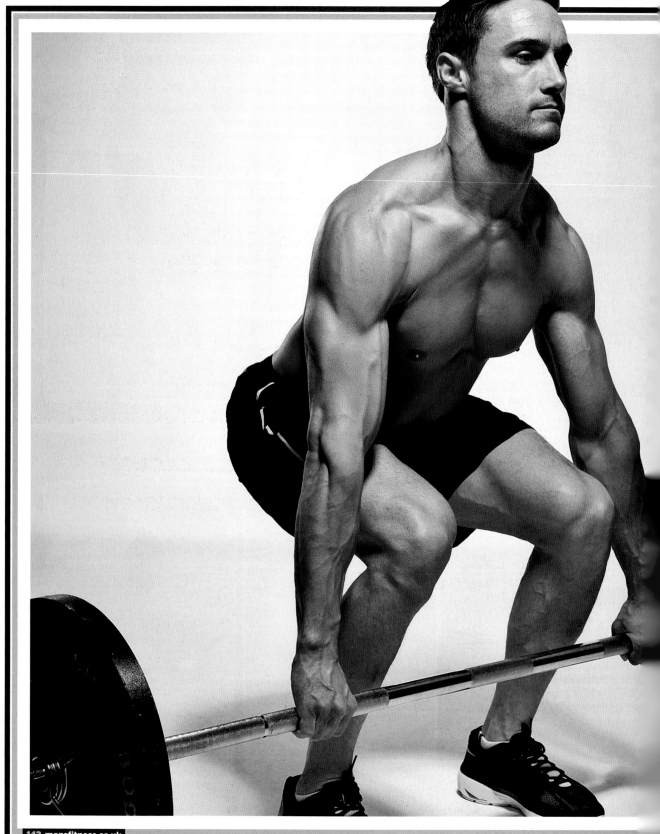

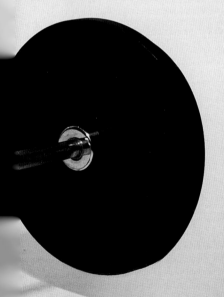

Total-body workouts

Work multiple muscle groups
to add bulk all over and
burn fat for a ripped look

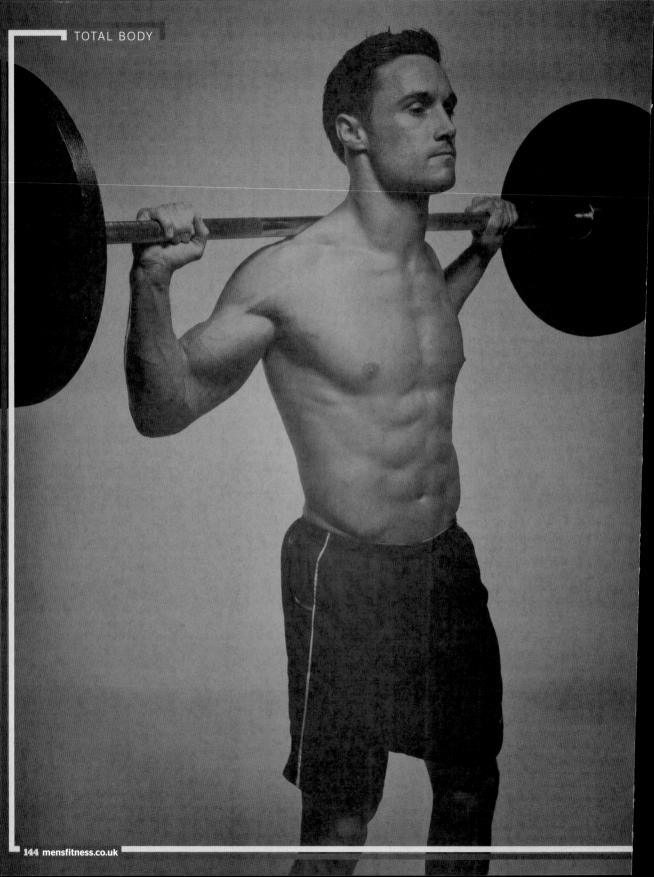

Total body blitz

One of the best ways to get into cover model shape is to perform full-body exercises. Making your muscles move as a single unit not only improves balance, co-ordination and power – all of which have huge transferable value to everyday life – but it is also one of the best ways to build muscle and burn fat. That's why the following four workouts include the major compound lifts in addition to muscle-specific isolation moves to blast your body into its best ever shape.

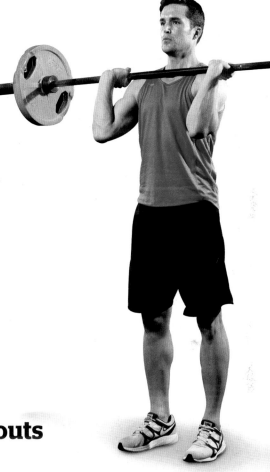

How to do the workouts

Make gains fast with these four total-body training plans

There are four workouts in this chapter. Each of these programmes is based on doing three sessions per week for a total of four weeks.

The first plan is a foundation workout designed for men of all athletic abilities, so make sure you start off by following this one rather than jumping straight into one of the three main workouts.

For those of you new to this type of exercise it will build a solid base from which you can launch into the more intense workouts. And even if you are a more experienced trainer, there's still much to gain from starting with the basics. It will help correct any muscular imbalances you may have, allow you to correct any poor form habits you may have picked up and let you master some simple movement patterns, including bodyweight moves, that you may have neglected during most of your previous training regimes.

Foundation workout

This workout prepares your entire muscular system to work together as a single unit so that you'll be able to attack the later workouts with good technique right from the get-go. Training your body to function efficiently as one is vital for not just building muscle and burning fat, but also for preventing injury and muscular imbalances.

EXERCISE		WEEK	REPS	SETS	TEMPO	REST
SUPERSET 1						
1a Press-up burpee		1 2 3 4	10 12 10 12	2 2 3 3	X X X X	
1b Dumbbell squat to press		1 2 3 4	10 12 10 12	2 2 3 3	2010 2010 2010 2010	90sec after 1b 90sec after 1b 90sec after 1b 90sec after 1b
SUPERSET 2						
2a Jump lunge		1 2 3 4	10 12 10 12	2 2 3 3	X X X X	
2b Bench dip		1 2 3 4	10 12 10 12	2 2 3 3	20X0 20X0 30X0 30X0	90sec after 2b 90sec after 2b 90sec after 2b 90sec after 2b
SUPERSET 3						
3a Dumbbell hammer curl		1 2 3 4	12 10 12 10	2 2 3 3	2010 2010 2010 2010	
3b Plank		1 2 3 4	1 1 1 1	2 2 3 3	20sec 30sec 20sec 30sec	90sec after 3b 90sec after 3b 90sec after 3b 90sec after 3b

1a Press-up burpee

TARGETS
Total body

WHY DO IT?
This is a great move for working multiple muscle groups at once and for getting your heart rate soaring.

HOW TO DO IT
● Start standing with your arms fully extended above your head, then squat down.
● As you reach the bottom of the squat, put your hands on the ground in front of you and kick your legs backwards until you are in a press-up position.
● Perform a press-up, then bring your legs back underneath you and jump up off the ground.

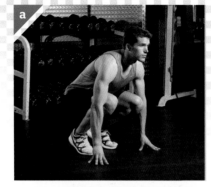

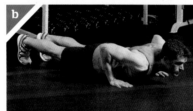

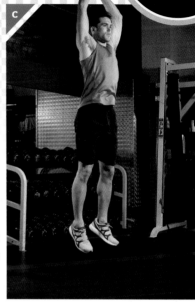

1b Dumbbell squat to press

TARGETS
Legs, core, shoulders

WHY DO IT?
It works most of your major muscle groups to promote a good growth-hormone response.

HOW TO DO IT
● Stand tall holding a dumbbell in each hand at shoulder height.
● Squat down, keeping your core braced, then stand back up and press the weights directly above your head.
● Reverse the entire movement back to the start.

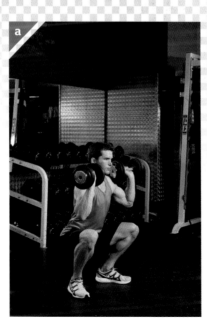

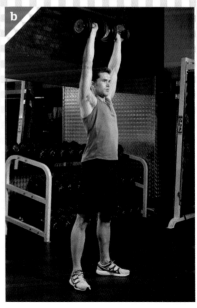

2a Jump lunge

TARGETS
Quads, hams, glutes, calves, core

WHY DO IT?
These require explosive power to jump high enough to switch legs and land straight back into a lunge, leading to rapid muscle growth and huge transferable value to many sports.

HOW TO DO IT
● Start in a lunge, then jump straight up.
● Switch legs in mid-air to land with your other foot forward.
● Descend straight into a lunge and repeat.

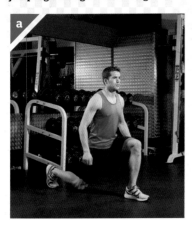
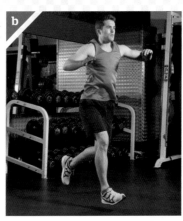
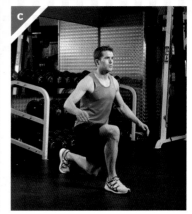

2b Bench dip

TARGETS
Triceps

WHY DO IT?
Build mass on the back of your arms with this surprisingly tough move.

HOW TO DO IT
● Place your hands on the edge of a bench behind you with your back and legs straight.
● Slowly lower your body straight down, keeping your elbows pointing back throughout, then press back up powerfully.

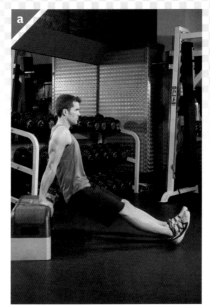
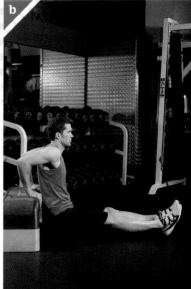

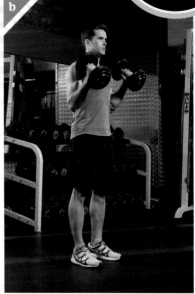
3a Dumbbell hammer curl

TARGETS
Biceps

WHY DO IT?

This move shifts some of the emphasis to the forearms so you work the muscles responsible for grip strength as well as your biceps. A stronger grip will help you in almost every other lift.

HOW TO DO IT

- Stand tall with your shoulders back and feet close together, holding a dumbbell in each hand with your palms facing each other.
- Keeping your elbows close to your sides, slowly raise the dumbbells to shoulder height, squeezing your biceps at the top of the move.
- Slowly return the weight to the start position and repeat with your other arm.

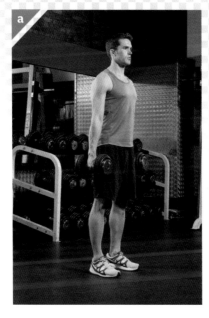

3b Plank

TARGETS
Core

WHY DO IT?

It builds a strong link between your upper and lower body.

HOW TO DO IT

- Hold your body in a straight line from head to heels with your elbows beneath your shoulders, feet together and head looking down.
- Hold the position for as long as you can without letting your hips sag.

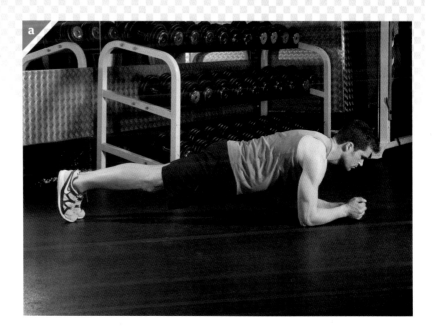

Workout one

This is a tough workout that will test all your major muscle groups in quick succession. The good news is that this will raise your heart rate so that you burn more calories during and after your session, while also fatiguing the maximum number of muscle fibres, which will then grow back bigger and stronger.

EXERCISE		WEEK	REPS	SETS	TEMPO	REST
SUPERSET 1						
1a Clean		1	6	2	X	
		2	6	3	X	
		3	8	3	X	
		4	8	3	X	
1b Squat		1	10	2	20X0	90sec after 1b
		2	8	3	20X0	90sec after 1b
		3	8	3	30X0	90sec after 1b
		4	8	3	40X0	90sec after 1b
SUPERSET 2						
2a Shoulder press		1	10	2	20X0	
		2	8	3	20X0	
		3	8	3	30X0	
		4	10	3	30X0	
2b EZ-bar biceps curl		1	12	2	20X0	90sec after 2b
		2	10	3	20X0	90sec after 2b
		3	12	3	30X0	90sec after 2b
		4	12	3	40X0	90sec after 2b
SUPERSET 3						
3a Close-grip bench press		1	10	2	20X0	
		2	8	3	20X0	
		3	8	3	30X0	
		4	10	3	30X0	
3b Cable woodchop		1	12	2	20X0	90sec after 3b
		2	10	3	20X0	90sec after 3b
		3	12	3	20X0	90sec after 3b
		4	12	3	30X0	90sec after 3b

1a Clean

TARGETS
Total body

WHY DO IT?
The clean involves almost all your major muscle groups and forces them to work together efficiently to move the bar as quickly as possible.

HOW TO DO IT
● Lift the bar off the ground by driving up through your heels.
● Once the bar reaches your hips, rise up on tiptoes, shrug your shoulders powerfully and pull it up onto the front of your shoulders.
● Return to the start.

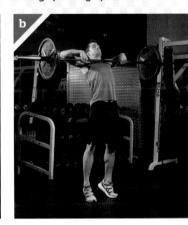
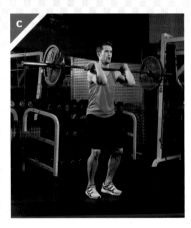

1b Squat

TARGETS
Quads, glutes, hamstrings, core

WHY DO IT?
Squats create an anabolic (muscle-building) state that triggers the release of extra testosterone and growth hormone in the bloodstream.

HOW TO DO IT
● Rest the bar against the back of your shoulders, holding it with an overhand grip.
● Your feet should be just wider than shoulder-width apart with your toes pointing outwards.
● Squat down until your thighs are at least parallel to the floor. The deeper you can squat, the better.
● Drive back up through your heels.

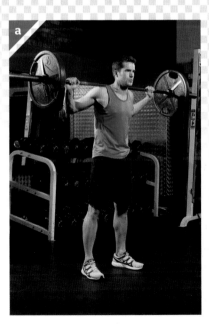
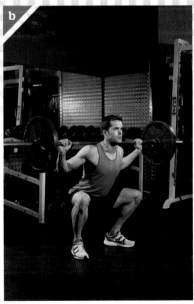

2a Shoulder press

TARGETS
Shoulders, triceps, core

WHY DO IT?
It mainly works the front and middle deltoids – two of the three major muscles that make up your shoulders – but also recruits your core.

HOW TO DO IT
● Hold a barbell across the front of your shoulders.
● Keep your chest upright and your core muscles braced.
● Press the bar directly upwards until your arms are extended overhead.
● Lower the bar back to your chest and repeat.

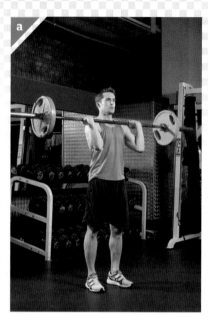
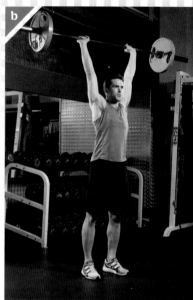

2b EZ-bar curl

TARGETS
Biceps

WHY DO IT?
An EZ-bar takes some of the strain off your wrists and allows the focus of the weight to be solely on your biceps.

HOW TO DO IT
● Stand tall with your shoulders back and feet close together, holding an EZ-bar with an underhand grip with hands just outside your hips.
● Keeping your elbows tucked in to your sides, curl the bar up towards your chest, stopping just before your forearms reach vertical.
● Lower back slowly to the start.

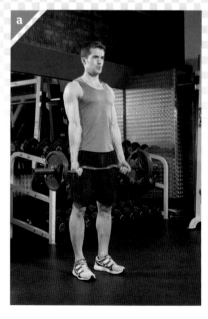
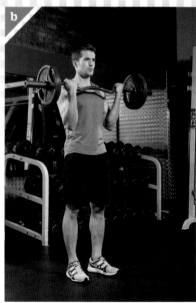

3a Close-grip bench press

TARGETS
Triceps, chest

WHY DO IT?
Bringing your hands closer together transfers the focus on to the triceps.

HOW TO DO IT
● Lie flat on a bench holding a barbell with a close, overhand grip.
● Lower the bar slowly to your chest, keeping your elbows close your sides.
● Push back up powerfully.

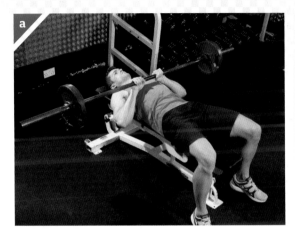
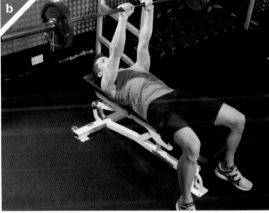

3b Cable rotation

TARGETS
Abs, obliques

WHY DO IT?
It's a great move to activate your entire core region.

HOW TO DO IT
● Attach an attachment to the middle of a cable stack.
● Standing next to it with a slight bend in your knees, back neutral, core braced and arms fully extended holding the handle with both hands, rotate your to move your arms across your body.
● Return slowly to the start.

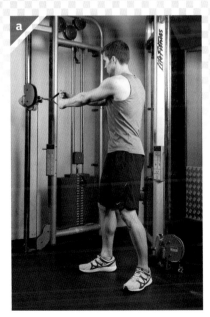
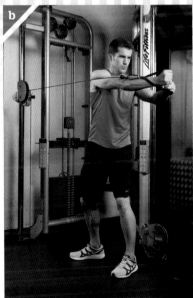

Workout two

Two hardcore supersets kick off this session, meaning your legs, core, back, chest and arms will all get a good workout in the most efficient and effective way. It finishes with moves to widen your shoulders and carve a six-pack, so no stone is left unturned.

EXERCISE		WEEK	REPS	SETS	TEMPO	REST
SUPERSET 1						
1a Clean and jerk		1 2 3 4	8 6 8 6	2 3 3 4	X X X X	
1b Bench press		1 2 3 4	12 10 12 10	2 3 3 4	30X0 30X0 30X0 30X0	90sec after 1b 90sec after 1b 90sec after 1b 90sec after 1b
SUPERSET 2						
2a Barbell lunge		1 2 3 4	12 10 12 10	2 3 3 4	20X0 20X0 20X0 20X0	
2b Pull-up		1 2 3 4	8 6 6 6	2 3 3 4	30X0 30X0 40X0 40X0	90sec after 2b 90sec after 2b 90sec after 2b 90sec after 2b
SUPERSET 3						
3a Lateral raise		1 2 3 4	12 10 12 12	2 3 3 4	2111 2111 2111 2111	
3b Plank		1 2 3 4	1 1 1 1	2 3 3 4	30sec 30sec 45sec 45sec	90sec after 3b 90sec after 3b 90sec after 3b 90sec after 3b

1a Clean and jerk

TARGETS
Total body

WHY DO IT?
It works all your major muscles to add size.

HOW TO DO IT
● Squat down and grasp the bar, then lift it by driving up through your heels.
● Once the bar reaches your hips, rise up on tiptoes, shrug your shoulders powerfully and pull the bar up, leading with your elbows.
● Squat back down under the bar and rotate your elbows forward to catch it on your shoulders.
● Squat down, then push up powerfully while driving your arms up directly above you.
● Return to the start.

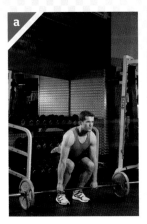
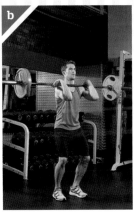
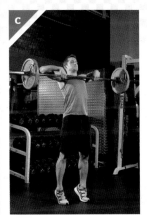
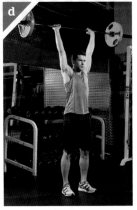

1b Bench press

WHY DO IT?
This classic lift also recruits the muscles at the front of the shoulders and back of the arms, making it a firm favourite for those wanting a big, strong torso.

HOW TO DO IT
● Start with your core braced, your back straight and your shoulder blades retracted.
● Bend your knees slightly and lean forward from the hips.
● Grip the bar with your hands just wider than shoulder-width apart letting them hang at knee level.
● Pull the bar up to your lower sternum, retracting your shoulder blades to allow the bar to come up to the chest, then lower the bar slowly to the start.

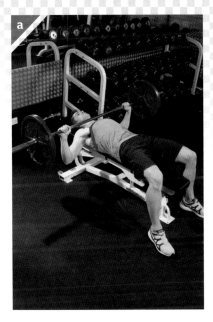
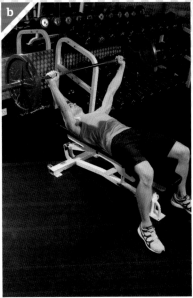

2a Barbell lunge

TARGETS
Hams, glutes

WHY DO IT?
Lunges work the glutes, quads, hamstrings and calves, but also involve the adductors, hip flexors and many other stabilising muscles – including your core.

HOW TO DO IT
● Stand tall with a barbell resting on the backs of your shoulders. Point your elbows behind you to retract your shoulder blades and keep your back upright and core braced throughout.
● Take a big step forward, making sure your knee does not go beyond your front foot. Lower down until both knees are bent at 90˚ before pushing off your front foot to return to the start position.

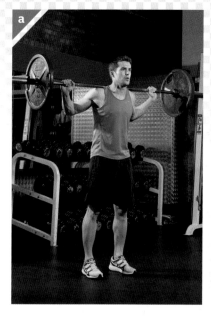
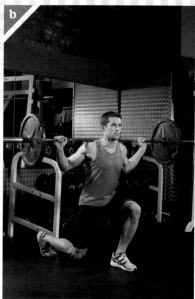

2b Pull-up

TARGETS
Upper back, core

WHY DO IT?
It builds a strong, wide upper back, which helps create the V-shaped torso that women usually love. Preventing your legs from swinging to work your core.

HOW TO DO IT
● Grab the bars with an overhand grip. If using a straight bar your hands should be slightly wider than shoulder-width apart.
● Start from a dead hang with your arms fully extended.
● Pull yourself up by squeezing your lats together.
● Once your chin is higher than your hands pause briefly, then slowly lower yourself back to the start.

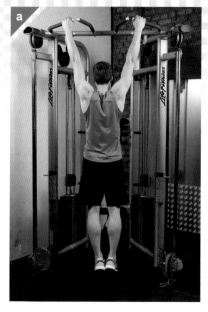
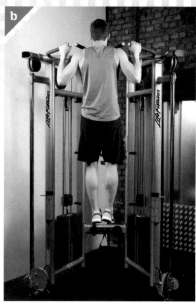

3a Lateral raise

TARGETS
Shoulders

WHY DO IT?
The lateral raise is one of the best moves at isolating the deltoids, especially those on the sides of your upper arms.

HOW TO DO IT
● Stand tall with core braced and feet apart, holding a light dumbbell in each hand by your sides with palms facing each other.
● Keeping a slight bend in your elbows, raise the weights out to the sides, using your muscles and not momentum.
● Stop at shoulder height, pause for a second, then lower slowly.

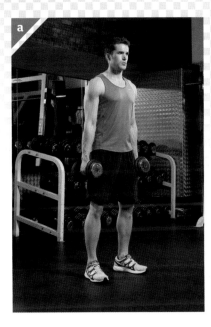
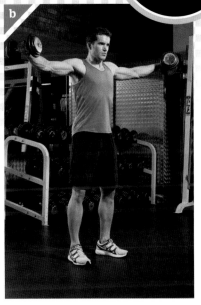

3b Plank

TARGETS
Core

WHY DO IT?
Nothing works your entire abdominal region as hard in such a short amount of time as the plank.

HOW TO DO IT
● Hold your body in a straight line from head to heels with your elbows beneath your shoulders, feet together and head looking down.
● Hold the position without letting your hips sag.

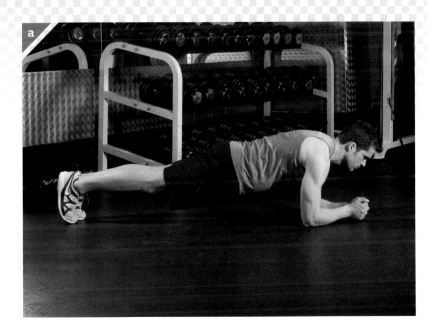

Workout three

The final total-body workout begins with the best moves for developing strong legs, lower back and triceps, then moves quickly on to target the upper back and biceps to create a V-shaped torso and big arms. Finally, the lower back and abs get a good going-over to ensure every last muscle gets some attention.

EXERCISE		WEEK	REPS	SETS	TEMPO	REST
SUPERSET 1						
1a Deadlift		1	6	3	20X0	
		2	8	3	20X0	
		3	6	4	20X0	
		4	8	4	20X0	
1b Triceps dip		1	8	3	30X0	90sec after 1b
		2	10	3	30X0	90sec after 1b
		3	8	4	30X0	90sec after 1b
		4	10	4	30X0	90sec after 1b
SUPERSET 2						
2a Lat pull-down		1	12	3	2111	
		2	10	3	2111	
		3	10	4	2111	
		4	12	4	2111	
2b Dumbbell squat to curl to press		1	12	3	2020	90sec after 2b
		2	10	3	2020	90sec after 2b
		3	10	4	2020	75sec after 2b
		4	12	4	2020	75sec after 2b
SUPERSET 3						
3a Gym ball back extension		1	12	3	2121	
		2	15	3	2121	
		3	12	4	2121	
		4	15	4	2121	
3b Crunch		1	12	3	2121	75sec after 3b
		2	15	3	2121	60sec after 3b
		3	12	4	2121	60sec after 3b
		4	15	4	2121	60sec after 3b

1a Deadlift

TARGETS
Total body

WHY DO IT?
It's perfect for developing a strong and supportive lower back, and because so many muscles are recruited you'll be able to lift a lot of weight.

HOW TO DO IT
● Grip the bar just outside your knees with your core braced, your shoulders retracted and over the bar and your back flat.
● Use your glutes to power the initial lift, pushing down through your heels.
● Keep the bar close to your body and, as it passes your knees, push your hips forward. Keep your shoulders back throughout the move.

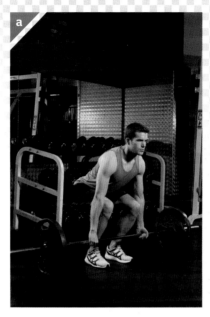
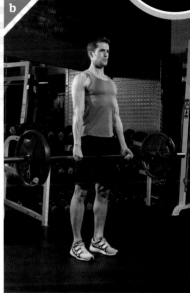

1b Triceps dip

TARGETS
Triceps, lower chest, shoulders

WHY DO IT?
The dip is one of the best moves to target all three parts of the triceps, as well as being great for working the lower chest, shoulders and your core, which you must keep tight to prevent your lower body swinging.

HOW TO DO IT
● Grip parallel bars, keeping your body upright.
● With your elbows pointing straight back, lower your body as far down as you can comfortably go without stressing your shoulders.
● Keep your core braced and don't swing your legs for momentum.

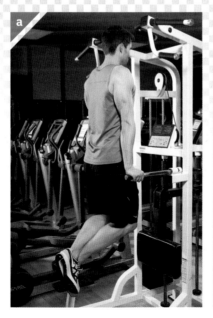
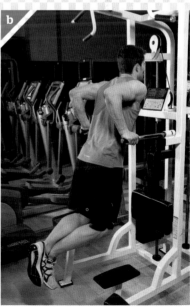

2a Lat pull-down

WHY DO IT?
This works the same muscles as the pull-up but the machine allows you to adjust the resistance more easily than a bodyweight move.

HOW TO DO IT
● Sit on the seat and take an overhand, wide grip on the bar.
● Look forward, retract your shoulder blades and keep your torso upright.
● Pull the bar down in front of you until it reaches your upper chest. Don't lean back to aid the movement.
● Squeeze your lats at the bottom of the move and return the bar slowly to the top.

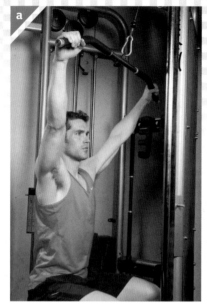
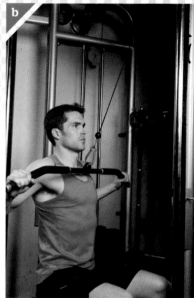

2b Dumbbell squat to curl to press

TARGETS
Legs, biceps, triceps, shoulders

WHY DO IT?
It works your major muscle groups, releasing growth hormone.

HOW TO DO IT
● Stand with a dumbbell in each hand, then brace your core and squat down.
● Stand back up, curling the weights up towards your shoulders, keeping your elbows close to your sides.
● From there, press the weights directly above your head then reverse the entire movement back to the start.

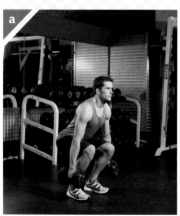
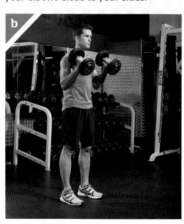
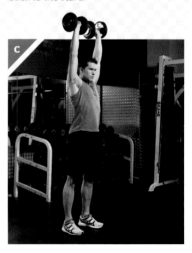

3a Gym ball back extension

TARGETS
Lower back

WHY DO IT?
You are only ever as strong as your weakest link and for most men it's their lower back.

HOW TO DO IT
- Lie over a gym ball with your hands by your temple.
- Raise your chest up and off the ball, pause at the top, then return slowly to the start.

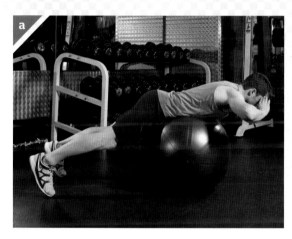
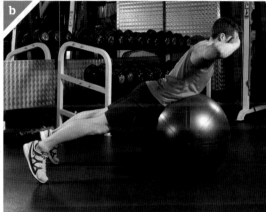

3b Crunch

TARGETS
Upper abs

WHY DO IT?
The classic move for targeting your upper abs.

HOW TO DO IT
- Lie with your back flat on a mat with knees bent at 90° and feet flat on the floor. Place your fingers by your temples.
- Contract your abs to lift your shoulders up and curl your chest towards your knees.
- Pause at the top of the move and squeeze your abs, then lower slowly to the start.

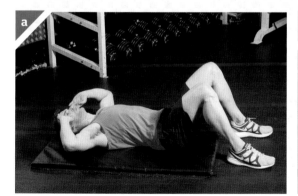
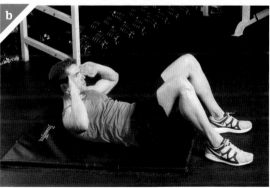

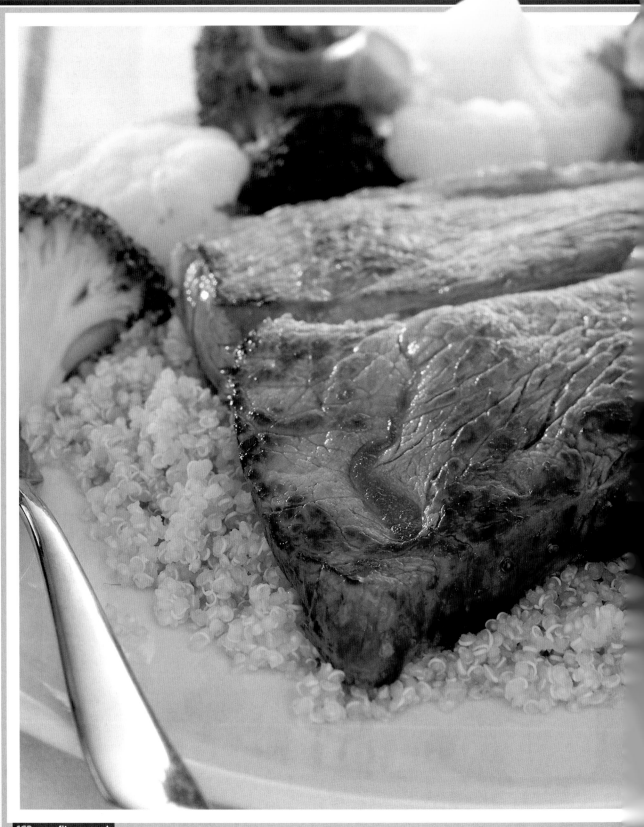

Eat for muscle

The food rules and supplements for building your cover model physique

The new rules of food

Eating properly shouldn't take a diploma, so we've condensed everything you need to know into seven simple rules

What you eat is every bit as important to your fitness as what you do in the gym and just as simple to follow. Here, we've distilled that collective wisdom into seven rules simple enough to scribble on a postcard. Memorise them, take them shopping or stick them on the fridge – and tuck in.

1 Green is good

THERE'S NO SUCH THING AS too much veg, especially if you're talking about vegetables grown above ground. Regardless of what else you're eating, your plate should be about half-full of them.

The Food Standards Agency's 'eatwell plate', which has replaced the traditional food pyramid as the government-endorsed illustration of what to eat, suggests that roughly a third of your diet should come from fruit and veg. But it also suggests that another third should be made up of 'bread, rice, potatoes and other starchy foods'.

This is not the way to a hard, lean body, because the fundamental problem with starchy carbohydrates is they cause sudden and prolonged rises in blood sugar, which is known to provoke a slew of biochemical imbalances that predispose you to weight gain, type 2 diabetes and other nasty health problems.

Besides, there's nothing in them that you can't get elsewhere. If you're going to eat carbohydrate, make sure it's more nutritious carbohydrate with slower sugar release, which is almost every vegetable apart from the potato.

It's also a bit of an oversimplification to put fruit and vegetables together, as the FSA plate does. Yes, they're both good for you, but they're radically different nutritionally. If you're getting your five a day alone from fruit, then your blood sugar levels are going to be going crazy throughout the day from the high fructose content.

If you want to get lean to show off your abs then it's worth remembering that you'd have to eat half a kilo of asparagus to ingest the same amount of carbs as you get in a single wholemeal pitta bread.

BITE-SIZED SUMMARY
Make vegetables the foundation of your diet, along with two pieces of fruit a day. Vary them as much as you can.

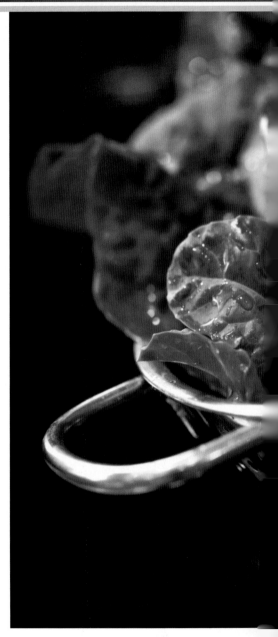

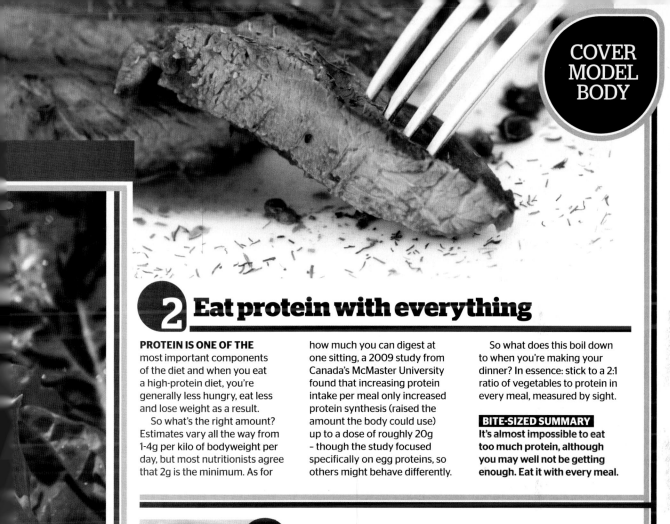

2 Eat protein with everything

PROTEIN IS ONE OF THE most important components of the diet and when you eat a high-protein diet, you're generally less hungry, eat less and lose weight as a result.

So what's the right amount? Estimates vary all the way from 1-4g per kilo of bodyweight per day, but most nutritionists agree that 2g is the minimum. As for

how much you can digest at one sitting, a 2009 study from Canada's McMaster University found that increasing protein intake per meal only increased protein synthesis (raised the amount the body could use) up to a dose of roughly 20g – though the study focused specifically on egg proteins, so others might behave differently.

So what does this boil down to when you're making your dinner? In essence: stick to a 2:1 ratio of vegetables to protein in every meal, measured by sight.

BITE-SIZED SUMMARY
It's almost impossible to eat too much protein, although you may well not be getting enough. Eat it with every meal.

3 Start as you mean to go on

YOU ALWAYS EAT BREAKFAST because you know it's the most important meal of the day and that skipping it slows your metabolism to a crawl. But are you still getting it wrong? You will be if you listen to the FSA's recommendation that you 'base your breakfast on bread or breakfast cereals' and 'wash it down with some fruit juice'.

Eating a high-carb breakfast will give you low blood sugar by mid-morning, making you more likely to snack on high-carb foods, which creates a vicious circle of snacking. So instead of starting your day with toast or cereal, have

something low-carb that's more nutritionally sustainable such as a plain full-fat yoghurt with berries and nuts or scrambled eggs with smoked salmon or ham.

Alternatively, just see off whatever's in the kitchen because last night's leftovers are one of the best (and cheapest) things you can eat, assuming you're eating right in the first place.

BITE-SIZED SUMMARY
Breakfast is like any other meal: you need protein, fats and fruit or veg. And there's no law stopping you from eating curry.

4 Calories don't count

CALORIES ARE NOT A GOOD indication of what a food is like and the effect it's going to have on your metabolic rate. Not convinced? Think of it this way: would you say that a couple of poached eggs are the same as a can of Coke because they contain a similar amount of calories? No.

Also, counting calories makes it too easy to justify bad dietary decisions. Ever heard a friend say that they can eat what they want because they'll burn it off at the gym? They couldn't be more wrong. In fact, the more active you are, the better your nutrition needs to be.

Arguably more important than calorie content is your food's glycaemic load (GL), which indicates how much of a blood sugar spike it'll give you – but manufacturers aren't required to put glycaemic load on the packaging. But if you're taking nutrition seriously that shouldn't be a problem. Steering clear of starchy food and sugar means you are already avoiding foods with high GL anyway.

You can also slow the absorption rate of high-GL foods, thereby helping prevent blood sugar wobbles, by eating them with protein-heavy foods such as chicken or tuna.

BITE-SIZED SUMMARY
Think quality, not quantity. Eating nutritious food is much better than sticking rigidly to a 2,000-calorie-a-day limit that comes from toast and crisps.

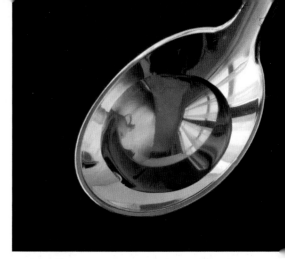

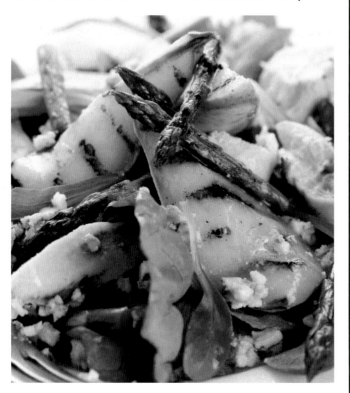

5 Don't fear fat

ALTHOUGH MOST OF US KNOW that eating some fat is essential to a healthy diet, it's all too easy to make a mental connection between eating fat and *getting* fat, so you end up simply avoiding it. The trouble is, that usually means eating something that's worse for you.

One possible issue the FSA has with fat is that it's more calorific, per gram, than carbohydrate or protein, but if you're worried about your weight one of the keys is to eat foods that are genuinely satisfying because you'll eat less of them, which is the case with high-fat foods. You also want to avoid spikes in insulin, which is what you're going to get if you eat a lot of carbs instead.

There's also the issue of whether it's OK to eat saturated fat – typically demonised as a cause of high cholesterol. Expert opinion is shifting towards the positive. The recent major reviews of the subject have not found a link between saturated fats and heart disease.

Hydrogenated and trans fats are a different story – the research there sounds alarm bells for fat storage – but there seems to be no cause for concern with naturally occurring fats such as those in red meat, avocado and nuts. After all, humans have evolved to eat saturated fats, so it seems strange that only in the last 50 years have they become bad for us. Grains, on the other hand, are a recent addition to our diets in evolutionary terms and may not be so easily processed by our bodies.

BITE-SIZED SUMMARY
Avoided partially hydrogenated fats, especially trans fats. Don't worry too much about the rest.

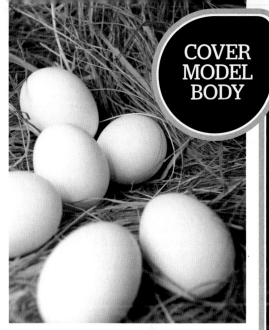

6 Free range is key

IN CASE THAT BULK-VALUE crate of cage-raised eggs is starting to look tempting, allow us to remind you favouring organic and free-range meat and fish is better for your body.

For instance, free range chickens have a more varied diet and a lot more exercise. This allows the development of more muscle and it also tends to contain more zinc, vitamins B, A and K, amino acids, iron, selenium, phosphorus and zinc.

Farm-raised salmon have been found to contain up to eight times the level of carcinogens as wild, thanks to cramped conditions and poor-quality feed, while grass-fed beef tends to have much more conjugated linoleic acid and omega 3s than the kind fed on grain and beef tallow. Think of it this way: free range is so nutritionally dissimilar to cage-reared that it's basically different food.

BITE-SIZED SUMMARY
Eat free-range chickens, grass-fed beef and wild-caught salmon when you can. If you don't know where it's from, chances are the answer isn't good.

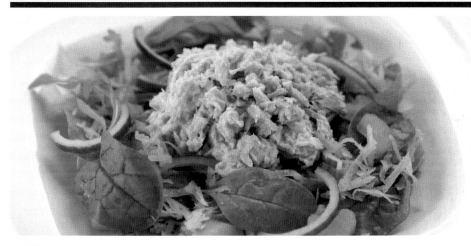

7 Eat real food

THIS IS THE KEY. If you do this, you'll end up following all the other rules almost by default. A simple rule of thumb is only eat food that grows out of the ground or food that once had a face.

Alternatively, simply go caveman and think like a hunter-gatherer. When you're looking at something on the shelf, ask yourself if it would have existed 5,000 years ago. If the answer is no, it probably isn't anything that you should be eating.

You may find it easier to stick to the 'right' aisles of the supermarket – you know, the ones with all the fresh veg, fruit and meat. You don't even need to go near the shelves that contain everything that's canned, processed or packed full of preservatives. Avoid things containing preservatives that you can't spell or ingredients you wouldn't keep in the kitchen. Eat things that will rot eventually, so that you know they're fresh. And try to enjoy it.

BITE-SIZED SUMMARY
Eat food, not products pretending to be food.

'A simple rule of thumb is only eat food that grows out of the ground or food that once had a face'

Cover model meal plan

Eat like a caveman to add strength and burn fat

For millions of years humans had no refined sugars or processed foods. So although such modern grub may be tasty and convenient, your body hasn't evolved to deal with it very well – and it usually encourages fat storage. This meal plan, created by nutritionist Christine Bailey (advancenutrition.co.uk) and based on the *Paleo Diet for Athletes*, replaces processed sugary foods and carbs with fresh fruit, nuts, seeds and animal proteins – the staple Stone Age foods. It has plenty of healthy unsaturated fats and branched-chain amino acids, which as well as aiding fat loss will help muscle development and anabolic function. If you're still peckish in the day grab a handful of nuts or drink a low-carb, high-protein shake.

42 PREHISTORIC MEALS TO KEEP THE FLAB AT BAY

MONDAY

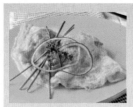

Breakfast
1 grapefruit. 2-egg omelette with ½ an avocado, spinach and 2 chopped tomatoes.

Snack
1 banana.

Lunch
150g grilled cod fillet with lemon juice and freshly ground black pepper. Green salad with lemon juice and 1tsp olive oil, 50g sugar snap peas, cucumber slices, ½ a red pepper and 2tbsp black olives. Bowl of blueberries and diced melon.

Snack
3 cold lean beef slices. Carrot sticks.

Dinner
Ginger baked turkey. 100g fresh raspberries with 2tbsp flaked almonds.

Snack
30g macadamia nuts. Handful of raisins.

DAILY TOTAL
1,840 calories, 163g carbs, 130g protein, 79g fat

TUESDAY

Breakfast
150g sautéed prawns with 6 sliced mushrooms and ½ chopped red pepper. 150g fresh pineapple slices.

Snack
Smoked salmon slices. Carrot and celery sticks.

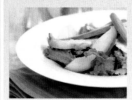

Lunch
Chicken and avocado salad. 1 apple. 30g almonds.

Snack
1 hard-boiled egg. 2 oatcakes.

Dinner
300ml home-made vegetable soup. Pan-fried venison with cherry sauce.

Snack
2 satsumas.

DAILY TOTAL
1,713 calories, 147g carbs, 156g protein, 60g fat

WEDNESDAY

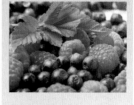

Breakfast
Bowl of blueberries and raspberries. 2 poached eggs with asparagus and 4 grilled mushrooms.

Snack
Handful of seeds. 1 apple.

Lunch
300ml home-made vegetable soup. Cold venison steak served with a bag of mixed salad leaves, ½ red pepper, 2tbsp black olives, sliced cucumber, celery and 1 tomato. Slices of melon.

Snack
2 slices of ham. Carrot sticks.

Dinner
Chicken and cashew nut stir-fry. Sliced fresh pineapple.

Snack
1 banana. Handful of macadamia nuts.

DAILY TOTAL
1,956 calories, 179g carbs, 130g protein, 87g fat

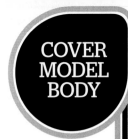

| THURSDAY | FRIDAY | SATURDAY | SUNDAY |

THURSDAY

Breakfast
Slices of melon with brazil nuts. 3 slices of lean roast beef with 2 baked tomatoes.

Snack
1 apple. Handful of raisins and almonds.

Lunch
300ml home-made vegetable soup. Grilled pork fillet with spinach salad (handful of baby spinach leaves, mixed lettuce leaves, ½ red onion, ½ red pepper, chopped fresh cucumber slices, celery). 1 satsuma.

Snack
1 hard-boiled egg. Carrot sticks.

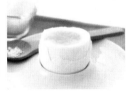

Dinner
Baked butternut squash and turkey casserole.

Snack
2 oatcakes. Smoked salmon slices.

DAILY TOTAL
1,841 calories, 201g carbs, 138g protein, 60g fat

FRIDAY

Breakfast
Bowl of cherries. 2 scrambled eggs with 5 asparagus spears.

Snack

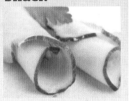

2 slices of ham, sliced cucumber and celery.

Lunch
Leftover squash and turkey casserole. Large mixed salad.

Snack
Handful of raisins and almonds. 1 pear.

Dinner
300ml home-made vegetable soup. Baked salmon fillet with lemon juice (cook an extra salmon fillet for Saturday) served with 60g steamed carrots, 60g sugar snap peas, 60g green beans and 1 baked sweet potato.

Snack
1 banana. Handful of cashew nuts.

DAILY TOTAL
1,816 calories, 185g carbs, 120g protein, 71g fat

SATURDAY

Breakfast
Bowl of blueberries and raspberries. 1 cold salmon fillet with pan-fried tomatoes and mushrooms.

Snack
4 oatcakes with ham.

Lunch
Grilled turkey breast with 1 baked sweet potato, salad leaves, cucumber, sugar snap peas, ½ a red pepper, 2tbsp black olives and ½ a red onion. Slices of fresh pineapple.

Snack

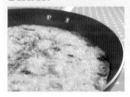

100g cooked prawns. Celery and carrot sticks.

Dinner
Frittata with 2 eggs, 3 new potatoes, spinach leaves, 1 red pepper. Steamed broccoli and carrots and salad.

Snack
1 banana. Handful of macadamia nuts.

DAILY TOTAL
1,827 calories, 172g carbs, 133g protein, 72g fat

SUNDAY

Breakfast
100g cooked prawns with green beans. 1 chopped apple and 2tbsp seeds.

Snack
2 slices of ham and 2 tomatoes.

Lunch
Lemon crab salad Slices of melon.

Snack
2 oatcakes. Smoked salmon slices.

Dinner
Pork stir fry. 1 satsuma.

Snack
2 oatcakes. Handful of almonds and raisins

DAILY TOTAL
1,746 calories, 159g carbs, 140g protein, 66g fat

Muscle-building snacks

Building post-workout muscle has never been easier or tastier

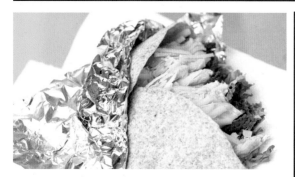

Recovery wrap

Building post-workout muscle has never been easier or tastier

Chicken and cheese wraps are a fast-food restaurant staple, but use your own fresh ingredients and they turn into superb muscle-building snacks. This grilled chicken wrap will help you to pack on bulk and recover faster after a testing workout.

What you will need

80g grilled chicken breast, shredded
1 wholemeal tortilla wrap
20g cheddar cheese, grated
30g cabbage, shredded

What you will get

Grilled chicken breast
As well as providing a large dose of lean protein vital for muscle growth and recovery, chicken also contains plenty of vitamin B3, which will help to prevent fat storage.

 Wholemeal tortilla wrap
A wholemeal tortilla wrap is packed full of carbs to help replenish your muscles, and it's also full of energy-boosting B vitamins.

 Cheddar cheese
This dairy product is a great source of casein, a high-quality muscle-protecting protein. It also contains high levels of bone-strengthening calcium.

 Cabbage
Cabbage is high in immune system-boosting vitamin C as well as plenty of dietary fibre, which your body needs to maintain a healthy digestive system.

Beef for bulk

Fuel your training with this tasty, meaty sandwich

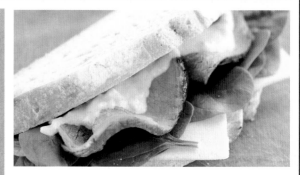

Eat this fitness-boosting snack an hour before your workout. Its quality carbs will give you the required energy for a tough session, while the protein helps you build muscle.

What you will need

2 thick slices of beef
2 thin slices of cheddar
2 slices of sourdough bread
Handful of spinach
1tsp of horseradish

What you will get

Beef
Beef contains high levels of slow-digesting protein – essential for muscle growth – and creatine, which increases muscle size by drawing water into your muscle cells.

Cheese
A source of casein, which is a high-quality muscle-building protein. The vitamin D in the beef also helps your body to absorb bone-strengthening calcium from the cheese.

Sourdough bread
Sourdough is low on the glycaemic index (GI), so it releases its energy slowly – more so than wholemeal bread.

Spinach
This is full of iron, which supplies working muscles with oxygen. It also contains betacarotene, an antioxidant that will soothe post-training stiffness and pains.

Horseradish
High levels of potassium help your muscles and nerves to function properly and lower your risk of high blood pressure.

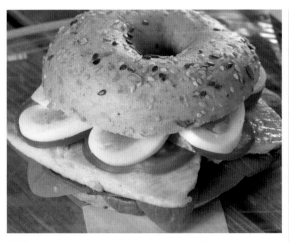

Energy bagel

This snack will fuel your training and help you build serious muscle

Snack on this before training and the carbs will help to keep your glycogen levels topped up, so your body doesn't have to use muscle-building protein as fuel.

What you will need

1 wholemeal bagel
2 thick slices of turkey
1 hard-boiled egg, sliced
1 sliced tomato
Handful of spinach

What you will get

Wholemeal bagel
A wholemeal bagel is packed with high-quality carbs for a sustained energy boost. It also helps contribute towards your daily requirement of dietary fibre.

Turkey
Turkey is a lean and low-calorie way to pack on muscle, thanks to its generous protein content. It is also rich in selenium, which strengthens the immune system and wards off the free-radical damage caused by exercise.

Egg
Eggs contain all the essential amino acids that your muscles need to build and repair themselves. They are also packed with testosterone-boosting zinc, which helps you to build muscle and burn fat.

Tomato
Vitamin C makes a hefty contribution to your amino acid metabolism, which helps the body to form new muscle. Tomatoes contain betacarotene and lycopene, which reduce inflammation and muscle soreness.

Spinach
Spinach is full of iron, which supplies working muscles with oxygen. Its high vitamin K content will also strengthen your bones.

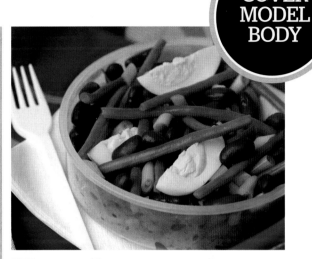

Two-bean muscle salad

You don't need meat for a protein-packed post-workout snack

Meat and fish aren't the only sources of protein. This vegetarian salad provides your body with protein to help you build muscle and recover faster after a hard workout.

What you will need

420g can red kidney beans, drained and rinsed
200g green beans
2 hard-boiled eggs, quartered
3 spring onions, chopped

What you will get

Kidney beans
A virtually fat-free source of high-quality, muscle-building protein, kidney beans are also rich in fibre, which keeps you feeling full for longer and is crucial for digestive health.

Green beans
One portion of green beans provides 25% of your daily vitamin K requirement, which helps to build strong bones. They're also a great source of both magnesium and potassium, which work together to help lower blood pressure.

Eggs
Eggs contain all the crucial amino acids that your muscles need to build and repair themselves. They're also packed with testosterone-boosting zinc, which is crucial to help you build muscle and burn fat.

Spring onions
The quercetin and vitamin C found in spring onions work in synergy to kill harmful bacteria and boost your immune system, while their high levels of chromium can help to keep blood sugar levels in check.

Bigger, stronger, faster

Supplements promise to help you get fit, lose fat and build a muscular physique – but do they work? And which ones do you really need? Here's all you need to know

Whether you regularly pack a protein shake in your gym bag or just chug the occasional isotonic sports drink, chances are you've used supplements at one time or another. Trouble is, the whole process can get a bit confusing – with every supplier claiming that its brand is better filtered, or more efficient, or will pack on more muscle – to the point where you feel like you need a degree in chemistry just to understand what you're putting into your body.

Don't worry – help is at hand. The science may be baffling, but we've put together the definitive guide that details all the latest developments in supplement science: what you need, when you need it, why you need it and what, if any, are the potential pitfalls.

You might find something that will send your training gains through the roof – or just learn more about the stuff you're already using. Either way, next time you put in a shift at the gym, you'll know that you're getting the nutritional backup you need.

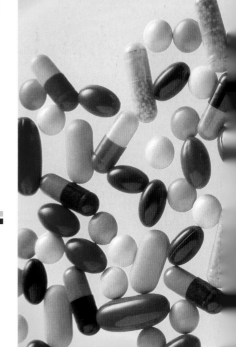

Protein

WHAT IS IT?
Protein is part of the structure of every cell and tissue in your body, and makes up around 20% of your bodyweight. It's needed to form new tissue as well as body enzymes and hormones.

WHAT DOES IT DO?
Protein is broken down for fuel during exercise, so you need a concentrated source of it to supplement your usual intake. Protein supplements ideally contain high levels of essential amino acids, which are readily absorbed by the body for muscle repair.

WHO SHOULD TAKE IT?
All athletes need to compensate for increased breakdown of protein during training. Strength athletes need extra to provide the stimulus for muscle growth.

HOW MUCH SHOULD I TAKE?
The Food Standards Authority recommends 55g of protein a day for adults, but most dieticians agree that this isn't enough if you're training regularly. The International Olympic Committee recommends 1.2-1.4g of protein per kilo of bodyweight a day for endurance athletes and 1.4-1.7g per kilo for power athletes.

HERE ARE THE BASICS
If you're below 10% body fat, try to have a post-workout shake with 0.6g of protein and 1.2g of carbs per kilo of lean bodyweight. So an 80kg man would need 43.2g of protein and 98.4g of carbs. If you're above 10% body fat then have the same amount of protein with the amino acids L-glycine and L-glutamine in place of carbs. But if you're a serious athlete then you can't really have too much protein – and any excess won't be stored as body fat. Unless you have a kidney disease, have as much as you like.

WHEN SHOULD I TAKE IT?
The most important thing is to make sure you get some protein early in the post-exercise recovery phase,

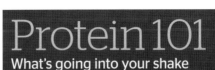
'Creatine is like a back-up generator for your body'

Protein 101
What's going into your shake

Casein

Casein, which makes up 80% of the protein content of milk, is made up of larger protein molecules, which are digested more slowly than whey, providing a slow, steady release of amino acids into the bloodstream. This slow release is what many experts argue makes it the best protein to use before going to sleep at night or for breakfast.

Whey

Whey, which is derived from milk, is digested and absorbed relatively quickly, making it useful for post-exercise recovery. It also has a higher concentration of essential amino acids than whole milk, which may help minimise muscle protein breakdown immediately after exercise.

Which is best after a workout?

Why not have both? What many people forget is that you can mix your whey with casein (milk) and get both. After a workout, if you mix a 25g scoop of protein powder into a 250ml serving of milk then you've got a big chunk of fast-acting whey right when you need it, with the all the added benefits of 16g of long-acting casein.

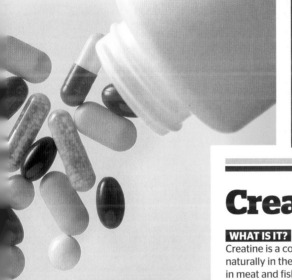

Creatine

WHAT IS IT?

Creatine is a compound that is made naturally in the body, but is also found in meat and fish or, in higher doses, supplements. It's available on its own and in some meal replacement shakes and other supplements.

WHAT DOES IT DO?

It's like a back-up generator for your body. Normally, energy in your body is produced, stored, and used via a chemical called adenosine triphosphate (ATP). But at times your body can't keep up with energy demand so it needs another source of phosphates, which is where creatine comes in. Creatine also helps promote the manufacture of protein and reduces its breakdown after exercise.

WHO SHOULD TAKE IT?

People who train with weights or do sports that involve repeated high-intensity movements, such as sprints, jumps or throws.

Bodybuilders often use it, because it increases muscle hypertrophy by drawing water into muscle cells.

HOW MUCH SHOULD I TAKE?

The average man takes in 1g of creatine a day from food and produces another 1g from amino acids, resulting in creatine stores that are about 40% below his maximum capacity. The best way to fill up is with doses of around 3g a day.

WHEN SHOULD I TAKE IT?

Avoid creatine before a workout because it draws water into your stomach and bloodstream, giving you cramps or a bloated feeling. The ideal time to take it is immediately after your workout.

ANY SIDE EFFECTS?

The main side effect is weight gain, partly because of increased muscle tissue but also because of the extra water in your muscle cells. There are some anecdotal reports of gastric discomfort, dehydration, muscle injury and kidney damage, but there is no clinical evidence to support these.

ideally immediately after exercise when your muscles need it most.

ANY SIDE EFFECTS?

It used to be thought that excess protein could damage the liver or kidneys, but this has only been demonstrated on those already suffering from kidney failure. High protein intake can potentially cause dehydration, but other than that it won't do you any harm.

Glossary

Here's what the fancy words on the label really mean

ANABOLISM

Anabolic processes build up organs and tissues, using smaller molecules to create larger ones. Anabolic steroids, for instance, increase protein synthesis in cells – although you'll see a lot of supplements that promise similar results without the side effects.

CATABOLISM

The breaking down of large molecules into smaller ones to produce energy. Products such as glutamine and antioxidants are said to reduce the rate of catabolism, so you'll recover from exercise faster.

HYDROPHILIC

Substances labelled hydrophilic dissolve easily in water or blood. Normal creatine, for instance, is hydrophilic, although you need to dilute it a lot.

LIPOPHILIC

Lipophilic substances pass through cell membranes easily, meaning they're absorbed quickly. Some expensive brands of creatine are more lipophilic than plain monohydrate, which they claim makes them more effective.

LOADING

Some lifters have to a 'loading' phase of supplement use, in which they take large amounts to build up stores. But if you take too much creatine or protein at once, your body just excretes it. Stick with the dose on the packet.

ION EXCHANGE

Ion exchange filtered protein has been separated via electrical charge. It means you'll lose some amino acids, but it also filters out a lot of fat and lactose.

MICROFILTRATION

Cross flow microfiltered protein uses a very fine membrane to filter proteins, leaving helpful amino acids intact, filtering out fat and leaving immune-boosting components untouched. It tends to be more expensive than ion-exchange-filtered protein.

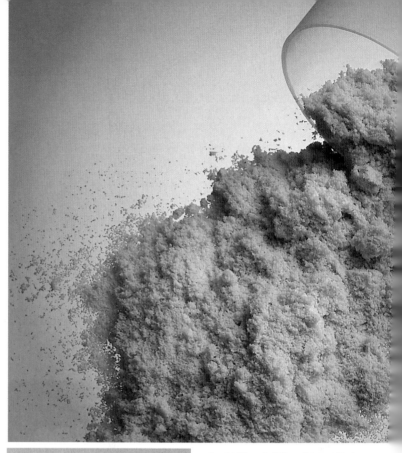

Amino acids

WHAT ARE THEY?

BCAA (branched-chain amino acids) supplements contain valine, leucine and isoleucine. These are 'essential' amino acids because they need to be present in your diet (your body produces 'non-essential' amino acids itself). Together, they can comprise up to one-third of muscle protein.

WHAT DO THEY DO?

They can help prevent the breakdown of muscle tissue during intense exercise. They also act to increase the release of human growth hormone.

WHO SHOULD TAKE THEM?

Anyone who's weight training. Opt for capsule form rather than tablet or liquid. There's little evidence that BCAAs will improve performance for endurance athletes.

HOW MUCH SHOULD I TAKE?

The science suggests that anything less than 20 capsules per workout is a waste of time. Many professional rugby and football clubs have seen huge improvements in performance using about 40 caps of BCAAs every workout.

WHEN SHOULD I TAKE THEM?

They work best if taken before, during and post-workout. Studies have shown that taking BCAA supplements taken before resistance training reduce delayed onset muscle soreness, while taking them during and after exercise can reduce muscle breakdown.

ANY SIDE EFFECTS?

BCAAs are fairly safe, since you'd normally find them in protein in your diet anyway. Too much might reduce the absorption of other amino acids.

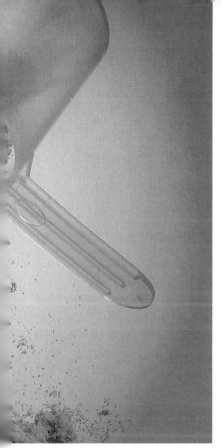

'Antioxidant supplements can protect against age-related diseases and cancer'

'Amino acids help prevent the breakdown of muscle tissue during exercise'

Anti-oxidants

WHAT ARE THEY?

Antioxidant supplements contain differing amounts of nutrients and plant extracts, including betacarotene, vitamins C and E, zinc, copper and magnesium. As well as having a beneficial effect on your general health, antioxidants can also help you recover from sports training.

WHAT DO THEY DO?

Very intense exercise can increase your body's generation of molecules known as free radicals, which can harm cell membranes, disrupt DNA and increase your risk of age-related diseases and cancer. Some evidence suggests that antioxidant supplements will protect against these diseases, though other studies suggest supplements are less effective than getting antioxidants as part of your diet. And there's not much evidence they'll actually help your sports performance.

WHO SHOULD TAKE THEM?

The jury is out but it has been suggested that, because of the environment and average stress levels, everyone should be on some type of antioxidant. They work best if rotated, so try having green tea and grapeseed extract on alternate days, for example.

HOW MUCH SHOULD I TAKE?

The EU recommended daily amount for vitamin C is 60mg and 10mg for vitamin E, but some scientists believe these levels are too low. Crucially, however, it's important to remember that supplements are no substitute for proper nutrition so aim to eat at least five portions of fruit and vegetables daily. Including as many different coloured fruits and vegetables as possible ensures you get the widest variety of antioxidants.

WHEN SHOULD I TAKE THEM?

This depends on the supplement you're taking and the effect you're looking for. Vitamin C is the antioxidant best taken after a workout because it blocks cortisol, the stress hormone. A 2008 study suggested that antioxidants are most beneficial when taken with meals – rats fed red wine alongside meat ended up with fewer free radicals in their digestive tracts than their non-drinking siblings – but the evidence isn't conclusive.

ANY SIDE EFFECTS?

There are side effects related to excessive consumption of certain vitamins found in antioxidant supplements – massive amounts of carotene can turn your skin temporarily orange, for example. Also, the antioxidant minerals zinc, magnesium and copper – can be toxic in large doses. If you stick to the recommended dosage, though, you'll be fine.

'Thermogenics can help you burn more calories'

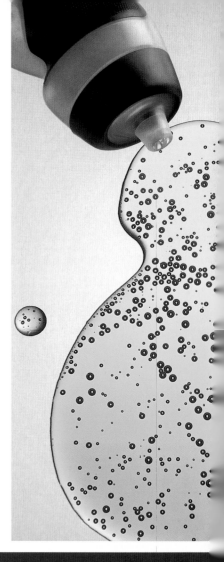

Fat burners

WHAT ARE THEY?

Also known as thermogenics, these are blends of herbs and stimulants that slightly increase your body temperature, which can help you burn more calories during exercise. Ephedrine used to be a key ingredient in these, but it's now only available on prescription in the UK due to its harmful side effects and addictive qualities.

WHAT DO THEY DO?

Some simply burn calories as heat. Others also claim to stimulate the release of adrenaline, increase your metabolic rate or act as appetite suppressants. The evidence for them working is limited, however, and a high-protein diet with regular exercise is likely to produce better weight-loss results in the long term.

WHO SHOULD TAKE THEM?

Fat burners raise cortisol – a stress hormone that in some cases may actually increase abdominal fat, especially if you're already leading a fairly stressful life. In extreme cases they can cause the adrenal system to get wiped out. If you think you need them consult your GP first.

HOW MUCH SHOULD I TAKE?

Follow the instructions on the bottle, but be careful with long-term use.

WHEN SHOULD I TAKE THEM?

Most contain caffeine and so will probably make you jittery, which means that the morning is the best time. Never take fat burners after 2pm because they affect sleep patterns, and always follow instructions on the bottle.

ANY SIDE EFFECTS?

Taking very high doses of ephedrine can have serious effects, including palpitations, anxiety, insomnia, vomiting and dizziness. While herbal alternatives are generally safer, you may get side effects with high doses – some can raise blood pressure or even cause heart disturbances.

What supp?

Your supplement queries answered

Can't my diet fulfil all my nutritional needs?

Yes, if you really watch what you eat, but sometimes you'll find that getting the optimum amount of certain substances means eating a lot. Getting all the creatine many trainers recommend would mean eating a mountain of beef. Use supplements to fill the gaps, but don't rely on them to counteract bad eating habits.

Do I need to take supplements on the days I'm not training?

Yes. You get stronger as you recover from exercise, so it's essential to get nutrients on your rest days.

Should I get up in the night to take supplements?

Almost definitely not. You might have heard about bodybuilders getting up at 3am to neck a quick shake, but as soon as you're awake for more than three seconds you disrupt the production of melatonin, one of the most important hormones in building muscle. You're better off having slow-digesting protein (raw nuts, cottage cheese or a casein shake) before bed.

Are they safe?

Since sports supplements are technically classified as food, they aren't subject to the same strict manufacturing, safety testing or labelling as licensed medicines so there's no guarantee that they'll live up to their claims. The EU is considering the introduction of stricter guidelines but it's currently up to individual manufacturers. Look for supplements that are ISO17025 certified, which means they've been subjected to rigorous checks during their production.

Can I fail a drugs test from taking supplements?

If you're a serious enough sportsman to be tested, then you need to be careful. A survey from an International Olympic Committee-accredited laboratory in Cologne studied 634 supplements and found that 15% of them contained

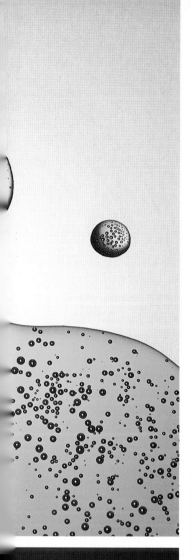

Best of the rest

What else is on the shelf of your local health food shop?

CLA

Conjugated linoleic acid is an unsaturated fatty acid normally found in full-fat milk, meat and cheese. It's usually marketed as a fat-loss supplement that works by releasing fat from fat cells or blocking new fat from getting in. Experts believe it's better at the latter and recent evidence suggests that CLA works mostly by inhibiting fat-cell filling, meaning it prevents fat cells from getting larger, which is not the same as causing loss of existing body fat. CLA may therefore turn out to be more useful for preventing fat gain than for causing loss of fat you already have. Most researchers recommend 2g-5g a day, divided into three doses.

Energy gels

These come in small squeezable sachets and are designed to provide an easy way of consuming carbohydrates during intense endurance exercise lasting longer than an hour. Studies have shown that they delay fatigue and increase endurance, but they aren't designed to do away with the need to carry water – you'll still need to drink around 350ml with every 25g of gel or you'll be at increased risk of dehydration.

HMB

Beta-hydroxy beta-methylbutyrate (HMB) is made in the body from BCAAs and is thought to be involved in cellular repair. Studies suggest that it may increase strength and muscle mass and reduce muscle damage after resistance exercise, although this hasn't been found in all studies. You can also find it in grapefruit.

Glutamine

Glutamine is a non-essential amino acid that the body synthesises. It is needed for cell growth and as fuel for the immune system. During periods of heavy training or stress, levels of it in the body fall. There's clinical evidence that glutamine supplements can decrease your risk of infection during these periods, but less evidence that it'll actually improve your performance.

MRPs

Meal replacement products are designed to provide the nutrients of a good-quality meal without the hassle of cooking. A good one will contain 30-40g of protein, some good carbohydrate sources such as maltodextrin, and vitamins and minerals. It's still better to eat fresh food if you've got the time, though.

Nitric oxide

The active ingredient in this is L-arginine, a non-essential amino acid made in the body. Nitric oxide is a gas involved in increasing blood flow to the muscles, delivering more nutrients and oxygen to them and theoretically causing a better pump, muscle growth and recovery. But, clinical trials haven't yet managed to prove that these supplements work.

Testosterone boosters

These aim to increase testosterone levels in the body, producing similar muscle-building effects to anabolic steroids without the side effects. There's plenty of anecdotal evidence to suggest that they work, but very little in the way of proven clinical trials.

ZMA

Zinc monomethionine aspartate combines zinc, magnesium, vitamin B6 and aspartate in a formula that claims to boost testosterone. If you're training intensely you might benefit from the extra zinc and magnesium but, as always, don't exceed maximum doses.

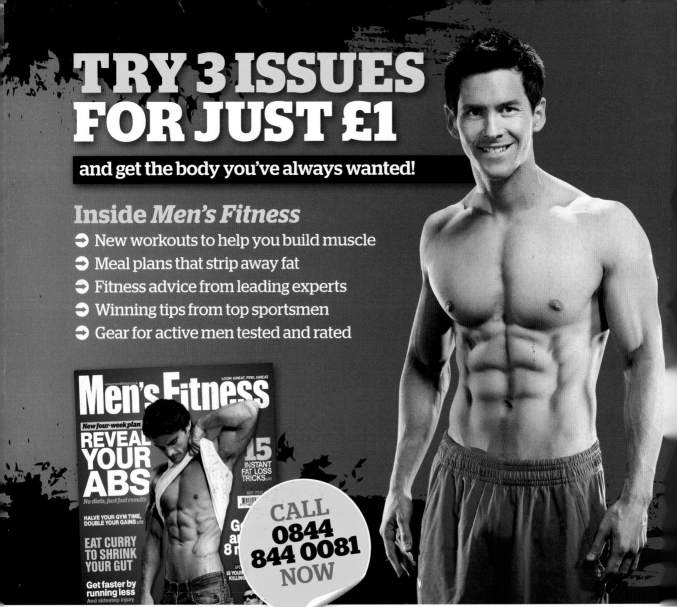